# A-Z
# SPORTS MEDICINE AND HEALTH MANAGEMENT

# A-Z SPORTS MEDICINE AND HEALTH MANAGEMENT

Dr. Aron Anisworth

CENTRUM PRESS
NEW DELHI-110002 (INDIA)

**CENTRUM PRESS**
**H.O.:** 4360/4, Ansari Road, Daryaganj,
New Delhi-110 002 (India)
Ph.: 23278000, 23261597

**B.O.:** No. 1015, Ist Main Road, BSK IIIrd Stage
IIIrd Phase, IIIrd Block,
Bangalore - 560 085 (India)
Tel.: 080-41723429
*Visit us at*: www.centrumpress.com

*A-Z Sports Medicine and Health Management*



First Edition, 2009

ISBN 978-93-80106-38-0

PRINTED IN INDIA

*Printed at* Salasar Imaging Systems, Delhi-110035 (India)

# Contents


| | | |
|---|---|---|
| | *Preface* | *vii* |
| 1. | Sports Medicine | 1 |
| 2. | Use and Abuse of Drugs in Sports | 32 |
| 3. | Central Nervous System Stimulants | 76 |
| 4. | Respiratory Tract Disorder Medicines | 122 |
| 5. | Androgenic Anabolic Steroids | 163 |
| 6. | Glycoprotein Hormones and Sport | 219 |
| 7. | Drug Treatment in Sports Injuries | 236 |
| 8. | Anti-anxiety Drugs and Sport | 275 |
| | *Index* | 311 |

# Preface

This title describes the turmoil seen in *Sports Medicine and Health Management* when blancing scientific, legal and ethical issue. Sports Medicine is defined not only by the customary definitation, but also by the issue surroundings the industry. Readers will gain a true appreciation for the complexity and intricacies of these issues that weave the tangled web of sports medicine. Readers will understand the background and history of Sports Medicine, legal and ethical issue and have new respect for everyone involved in the field.

*Sports Medicine and Health Management* specializes in preventing, diagnosing and treating injuries related to participating in sports and/or exercise, specifically the rotation or deformation of joints or muscles caused by engaging in such physical activities. The sports medicine "team" includes specialty physicians and surgeons, athletic trainers, physical therapists, coaches, other personnel, as well as the athlete himself/herself.

Sports medicine has always been difficult to define because it is not a single specialty, but an area that involves health care professionals, researchers and educators from a wide variety of disciplines. Its function is not only curative and rehabilitative, but especially preventive. Despite this wide scope, there has been a tendency for many to assume that sport-related problems are by default musculoskeletal and that sports medicine is an orthopaedic specialty.

Author

# Chapter 1

# Sports Medicine

## DEFINITION OF A DRUG

Drugs are chemical substances which, by interaction with biological targets, can alter the biochemical systems of the body. The branch of science investigating drug action is known as pharmacology. These interactions may be mediated through a variety of target tissues within the body. For example, effects on cardiac muscle by drugs such as ephedrine can lead to an increase in the force and rate of beating of the heart; stimulation of nerve endings in the central nervous system by drugs such as amphetamine can produce changes in mood and behaviour; interaction with metabolic processes, with drugs such as insulin, can be used in the treatment of disorders such as diabetes. Frequent reference is made to drugs on the International Olympic Committee (IOC) list of doping classes and methods.

## CLASSIFICATION AND DESCRIPTION OF DRUG NAMES

Drugs are variously classified and described by their:

- Generic name (international non-proprietary name: INN)
- Proprietary name
- Mechanism of action

The generic name (INN) is the internationally recognized name of the drug and should normally be used when describing the drug. When a pharmaceutical company first develops a new drug, it patents the drug under a proprietary name. When the patent expires, other pharmaceutical companies may produce the same drug but they give the drug their own proprietary name to distinguish their version of the drug from that of other companies.

**Table:** Examples of the classification and description of drugs by their names

| *Class of drug* | *Generic name* | *Proprietary names* |
|---|---|---|
| Androgenic anabolic steroids | Stanozolol<br>Nandrolone | Stromba<br>Deca-Durabolin |
| Diuretics | Furosamide | Lasix |
| β2 -Agonists (bronchodilators) | Salbutamol | Ventolin; Aerolin |
| Narcotic analgesics | Morphine | Oramorph; Sevredol |
| Beta blockers | Atenolol<br>Propranolol | Tenormin<br>Inderal |
| Human growth hormone | Somatropin | Genotropin; Humatrope |

**Table:** Classification of drugs and their use

| *Class of drug* | *Pharmacological action* | *Therapeutic use in:* |
|---|---|---|
| Diuretics | Prevention of reabsorption of water | Heart failure from the kidneys<br>Hypertension |
| β2 -Agonists | Bronchodilation through stimulation of β2-adrenoreceptors | Asthma<br>Chronic obstructive pulmonary disease |
| Aspirin | Inhibition of prostaglandin synthesis | Mild pain<br>Inflammation |
| | Reduction in platelet adhesion | Thrombotic diseases |
| Morphine | Agonist on opioid μ receptors | Severe pain |
| Beta blockers | Antagonists on β-adrenoreceptors | Angina Hypertension<br>Cardiac arrhythmias<br>Anxiety |

The mechanism of action describes the pharmacology of the drug and the therapeutic use for which the drug is designed. The mechanism of action of some commonly used drugs in terms of their pharmacological action and the therapeutic uses for which they are prescribed.

## DEVELOPMENT OF NEW DRUGS

Over the centuries, herbalists and apothecaries have experimented with potions derived from plant and animal sources. Indeed, some drugs are still derived from natural sources. For example, the morphine group of drugs is extracted from the fruiting head of the opium poppy and digoxin is derived from the foxglove plant. However, the majority of drugs are produced through chemical synthesis. The pharmaceutical industry is one of the largest and most successful international organizations. Companies are continually striving, through research and development, to produce new drugs. Current research into gene technology is likely to revolutionize the development of new drugs in the future.

The development of new drugs is monitored by government agencies who evaluate data on the activity and safety of new drugs before the company is awarded a product licence. In the USA the agency is the Food and Drug Administration (FDA), in the UK it is the Medicines Control Agency (MCA).

Agencies do not always agree, therefore a drug may have a product licence in one country but not in another. The product licence states the therapeutic purpose for which the drug may be used. This, again, may vary from one country to another. The development of new drugs can take between 10 and 12 years and cost several hundred million dollars.

### Dosage forms for Drug Delivery to the Body

There are many different dosage forms through which drugs can be delivered to particular sites in the body. Examples of dosage forms for drugs subject to restrictions in sport. The selection of the most appropriate dosage form depends on a number of factors:

- Speed of action
- Oral preparations are slow to be absorbed from the

gastrointestinal tract. Modified release tablets can slow this process even more, to give a longer duration of action.

- Injections, particularly intravenous, are very rapid.
- Aerosol inhalers provide rapid effects on the airways.
- Transdermal patches provide a slow sustained delivery by absorption through the skin.
- Site of action
- Oral and most injection preparations lead to extensive distribution of the drug around the body.
- Creams/ointments/ear drops/eye drops/aerosol inhalers are each delivered to the site where they are specifically needed.
- Reduction of side-effects
- Generally, the more widely distributed the drug is in the body, the greater the chance of side-effects. Therefore, topical administration has advantages over systemic delivery by mouth or by injection.

**Table:** Major routes of administration for drugs

| Route | Examples of dosage forms |
|---|---|
| Oral | Tablets, capsules, syrups |
| Buccal | Lozenges, sublingual (dissolved under the tongue) tablets, buccal sprays |
| Injections | Intravenous, intramuscular, subcutaneous, intra-articular (into a joint such as the knee) |
| Topical | Dermatological (creams, ointments, lotions, sprays) Drops (ear, eye, nose) |
| Inhalation | Aerosols, dry powders |
| Rectal | Suppositories |
| Vaginal | Pessaries |

## THE ABSORPTION, DISTRIBUTION, METABOLISM AND ELIMINATION OF DRUGS

For a drug to exert its effect it must reach its site of action. This will involve its passage from the site of administration to the cells of the target tissue or organ. The principal factors which can influence this process are absorption, distribution, metabolism and elimination. Consideration of these factors is known as the pharmacokinetics of drug action.

## Absorption

The absorption of a drug is, in part, dependent upon its route of administration. Most drugs must enter the bloodstream in order to reach their site of action and the most common route of administration for this purpose is orally, in either liquid or tablet form. Absorption from the gut can be affected by:

- Lipid solubility of the drug
- Gastrointestinal motility
- Gastrointestinal pH (acidity)
- Physicochemical interaction with the contents of the gut (enzymes, food, other drugs)

Where a drug is required to act more rapidly, or is susceptible to breakdown in the gastrointestinal tract, the preferred route of administration is by injection. There are a number of routes through which drugs are injected and the main ones are subcutaneous (under the skin), intramuscular (into a muscle) and intravenous (directly into the bloodstream via a vein).

Many drugs can be applied topically for a localized response. This may take the form of applying a cream, ointment or lotion to an area of skin IOC regulations regarding the route of administration for drugs which are subject to restrictions treatment of abrasions, lesions, infections or other such dermatological conditions. Topical applications may also involve applying drops to the eye, the ear or the nose. Drugs administered by a topical route are not normally absorbed into the body to the same extent as drugs administered orally. Consequently, the IOC regulations regarding certain drugs are complex.

## Distribution

Apart from topical administration, a significant proportion of a drug will reach the bloodstream. Most drugs are then dissolved in the water phase of the blood plasma.

Within this phase some of the drug molecules may be bound to proteins and thus may not be freely diffusible out of the plasma. This will affect the amount of drug reaching its target receptors. Plasma protein binding is but one factor in the complicated equation of drug distribution. As a general rule the amount of drug reaching its target tissue is a small proportion of the total drug in the body. Most of the drug remains in solution within the various fluid compartments of the body.

The principal fluid compartments are: the plasma, the interstitial spaces between the cells and the fluid within the cells of the body (intracellular). These compartments are separated by capillary walls and cell membranes, respectively. Therefore, drugs which can pass through the capillary wall but are unable to cross cell membranes are distributed in the extracellular space and those drugs which permeate all membranes are found within the total body water.

Very few molecules, with the exception of proteins, are unable to cross capillary walls; hence, most drugs, except those which extensively bind to plasma protein, can be found outside the plasma. For a drug to be able to penetrate cell membranes it must be lipid soluble as well as water soluble. The majority of drugs are lipid soluble and are therefore widely distributed throughout the total body water.

Drugs which are not lipid soluble are unable to penetrate the cells of the gastrointestinal tract and are therefore poorly absorbed orally. Such drugs must be administered by injection. An additional obstruction to the passage of drugs occurs at the 'blood-brain barrier' which comprises a layer of cells which covers the capillary walls of the vessels supplying the brain. This barrier effectively excludes molecules which are poorly lipid soluble. The blood-brain barrier is an important factor to be considered in drug design since a drug's ability to cross this barrier can influence its potential for centrally mediated side-effects.

## Metabolism

The body has a very efficient system for transforming

chemicals into safer molecules which can then be excreted by the various routes of elimination. This process is known as metabolism and many drugs which enter the body undergo metabolic change. There are several enzyme systems which are responsible for producing metabolic transformations. These enzymes are principally located in the cells of the liver but may also be found in other cells. They produce simple chemical alteration of the drug molecules by processes such as oxidation, reduction, hydrolysis, acetylation and alkylation. The consequences of drug metabolism may be seen in a number of ways:

- An active drug is changed into an inactive compound. This is a common metabolic process and is largely responsible for the termination of the activity of a drug.
- An active drug can be metabolized into another active compound. The metabolite may have the same pharmacological action as the parent drug or it may differ in terms of higher or lower potency or a different pharmacological effect.
- An active drug can be changed into a toxic metabolite.
- An inactive drug can be converted into pharmacologically active metabolites. This mechanism can occasionally be used for beneficial purposes where a drug is susceptible to rapid breakdown before it reaches its site of action. In this case a 'prodrug' can be synthesized which is resistant to breakdown, but which will be metabolized to the active drug on arrival at its target tissue.

Generally speaking, the metabolism of drugs results in the conversion of lipid-soluble drugs into more water-soluble metabolites. This change affects distribution, in that less lipid-soluble compounds are unable to penetrate cell membranes. The kidneys are able to excrete water-soluble compounds more readily than lipid-soluble molecules since the latter can be reabsorbed in the kidney tubules and therefore re-enter the plasma.

Metabolism is a very important factor in determining a

drug's activity since it can alter the drug's intrinsic activity, its ability to reach its site of action, and its rate of elimination from the body. Many drugs are completely metabolized before being excreted in the urine.

## THE IOC TESTING PROCEDURES IN DOPING CONTROL DETECT

### Elimination

There are many routes through which drugs can be eliminated from the body:

- Kidneys (urine)
- Salivary glands (saliva)
- Sweat glands (sweat)
- Pulmonary epithelium (exhaled gases)
- Mammary glands (mammary milk)
- Rectum (faeces)

Excretion via the rectum in the faeces may take place either by passage from the blood into the colon or through secretion with the bile.

The most important route for drug excretion, however, is through the kidneys into the urine. Most drugs and their metabolites are small molecules which are water soluble and as such can be easily filtered through the capillaries within the glomeruli of the kidneys. Having been filtered out from the plasma, the molecules may be reabsorbed, to a greater or lesser extent, from the renal tubules. This will depend on their lipid/water partition coefficients, and on whether there is a specific membrane carrier transport system for the particular molecule.

The net effect, in all cases, is that a constant fraction of the drug is eliminated at each passage of the blood through the kidney filtration system. The drug and/or its metabolites are then voided with the urine. It is for this reason that urine sampling is the principal method used in dope testing. The methods available for detecting drugs and their metabolites are extremely sensitive and capable of determining both the nature and the concentration of the drug/metabolite present.

Peptide hormones, which are synthesized in the body, have produced difficulties with regard to dope testing. At the time of writing, a suitable test for human growth hormone, acceptable to the IOC, had not been implemented, despite significant resources having been invested in developmental research.

On the other hand, an accredited testing system for erythropoietin (EPO) was introduced for the first time at the Sydney 2000 Olympic Games. The test comprised both a urine-based and a blood-based test and relied on the fact that EPO, used by athletes, is derived from recombinant DNA technology. This instils subtle differences in the properties of recombinant EPO (rEPO) compared with endogenous EPO, produced by the body. The urine test used electrophoretic techniques to distinguish between rEPO and EPO. The blood test identified characteristic changes in blood cell morphology, induced by rEPO.

Pharmacological means have been used in an attempt to mask drug-taking activities. These have included the concomitant use of drugs such as probenecid, whose therapeutic use is in the treatment of gout. Probenecid has also been used for many years in combination with certain antibiotics, as it will delay the excretion of these antibiotics and therefore prolong their antibacterial effect within the body. This property of probenecid has been used by competitors to try to delay the excretion of banned drugs such as anabolic steroids and thereby avoid detection. However, this effect is not absolute and the testing procedures are sophisticated enough to detect minute quantities of drugs in the urine. Probenecid itself has been on the IOC list of banned substances since 1987.

## EFFECT OF EXERCISE ON PHARMACOKINETICS

Under most circumstances exercise does not affect the pharmacokinetics of drug action. During severe or prolonged exercise, blood flow within the body will be altered, with a decrease in blood supply to the gastrointestinal tract and to the kidneys. However, there is little documentary evidence to suggest that such changes significantly affect the pharmacokinetics of the majority of drugs.

## Drugs and their Targets

Ideally, a drug should interact with a single target to produce the desired effect within the body. However, all drugs possess varying degrees of side-effects, largely dependent on the extent to which they interact with sites other than their primary target.

During their development, drugs undergo a rigorous evaluation in an endeavour to achieve maximum selectivity. The aim of selectivity is to increase the drug's ability to interact with those sites responsible for inducing the desired therapeutic effect whilst reducing the drug's tendency to interact with secondary target sites which are responsible for producing its side-effects.

Drugs can interact with enzymes, carrier molecules and ion channels in cell walls to produce their pharmacological effect. However, the sites through which most drug molecules interact are known as receptors.

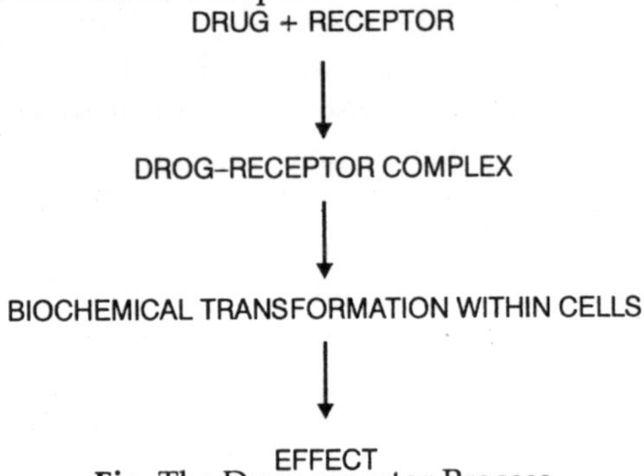


**Fig.** The Drug-receptor Process.

These receptors are normally specific areas within the structure of cells. They may be located intracellularly but most receptor sites are found on cell membranes. Receptors are present within cells to enable naturally occurring substances, such as neurotransmitters, to induce their biochemical and physiological functions within the body. We exploit the fact that receptors exist, by designing drugs to stimulate (agonists) or block (antagonists) these receptors and thereby intensify or reduce biochemical processes within the body.

The interaction between a drug (ligand) and a receptor is the first step in a series of events which eventually leads to a biological effect. The drug receptor interaction can therefore be thought of as a trigger mechanism.

There are many different receptor sites within the body, each of which possesses its own specific arrangement of recognition sites. Drugs are designed to interact with the recognition sites of particular receptors thereby inducing an effect in the tissue within which the receptors lie. The more closely a drug can fit into its recognition site the greater the triggering response and therefore the greater the potency of the drug on that tissue.

In designing drugs it is sometimes necessary to sacrifice some degree of potency on the target receptor site in order to decrease the drug's ability to interact on other receptors. A tendency towards the therapeutic effect and away from side-effects is thereby achieved, thus producing a greater degree of selectivity.

## AGONISTS AND ANTAGONISTS

A drug which mimics the action of an endogenous biochemical substance is said to be an agonist. The potency of agonists depends on two parameters:

- affinity- the ability to bind to receptors
- efficacy- the ability, once bound to the receptor, to initiate changes which lead to effects

Another group of drugs used in therapeutics is known as antagonists. They also have the ability to interact with receptor sites but, unlike agonists, do not trigger the series of events leading to a response. Their pharmacological effect is produced by preventing the body's own biochemical agents from interacting with the receptors and therefore inhibiting particular physiological processes.

A typical example of this can be seen with the group of drugs known as the beta blockers. They exert their pharmacological and therapeutic effects

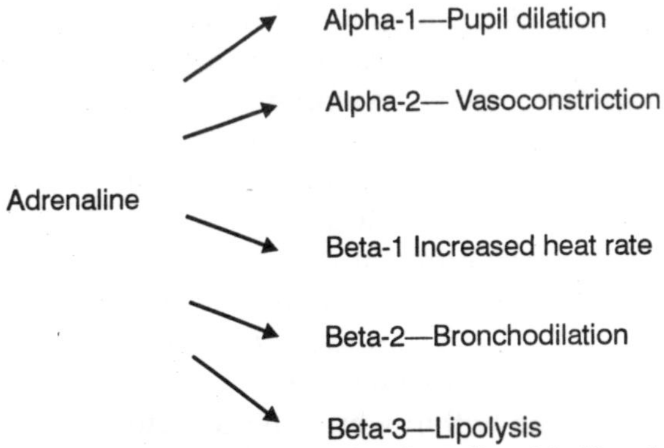


**Fig.** Some Physiological Effects of Adrenaline Mediated through the five Principal Classes of Adrenergic Receptors.

by occupying beta receptors without stimulating a response but, by so doing, prevent the neurotransmitter noradrenaline (norepinephrine) and the hormone adrenaline (epinephrine) from interacting with these receptors. One of the physiological functions mediated by noradrenaline and adrenaline through beta receptors is to increase heart rate in response to exercise or stress, therefore the administration of a beta blocker antagonizes this effect thereby maintaining a lower heart rate under stress conditions.

The principle of drug selectivity applies equally to agonists and antagonists. Research into drug-receptor interactions has led to a greater understanding of receptor structure and function, consequently, the original concepts of receptors have had to be modified. There are now many examples of receptor subclassification allowing for a greater degree of selectivity in drug design.

This can be illustrated by looking at the effect of adrenaline (epinephrine) on adrenergic receptors. We know that there are at least five subclasses of adrenergic receptors, known as alpha-1 ($\alpha 1$) alpha-2 ($\alpha 2$) beta-1 ($\beta 1$) beta-2 ($\beta 2$) and beta-3 ($\beta 3$). Adrenaline can interact with all of these receptors producing a variety of physiological effects. The drug called salbutamol was developed to have a selective effect on $\beta 2$ - receptors. It therefore produces bronchodilation, without the other effects associated with adrenaline. As such it is a first-line drug in the treatment of asthma. The selective nature of salbutamol is recognized by the IOC who permit its use in sport whilst other less selective sympathomimetics are banned.

## Side-effects of drugs

It is important to remember that all drugs, even the most selective, produce side-effects. For patients taking drugs for therapeutic purposes, these side-effects may be deemed acceptable when weighed against the beneficial therapeutic effects of the drug. However, no such counterbalance exists for individuals, such as athletes, taking drugs for nontherapeutic purposes. In this case, side-effects can only be perceived as detrimental to health.

***Table:*** Side-effects associated with some drugs that are commonly misused in sport

| *Class of drugs* | *Side-effects* |
|---|---|
| Amphetamines | Restlessness; irritability; tremor; insomnia; cardiac arrhythmias; aggression; addiction. |
| β2 -Agonists | Tremor; tachycardia; cardiac arrhythmias; insomnia; headache |
| Narcotic analgesics | Constipation; respiratory depression; addiction |
| Anabolic androgenic steroids | Acne; hypertension; mania; depression; aggression; liver and kidney tumours |
| | In females: masculinization; cliteromegaly |
| | In males: testicular atrophy; gynaecomastasia |
| Diuretics | Dehydration; muscular cramp |
| Human growth hormone | In children: gigantism |
| | In adults: acromegaly (hypertension; diabetes; muscular weakness; thickening of the skin) |
| Erythropoietin | Flu-like symptoms; hypertension; thromboses |

Some side-effects to drugs occur at normal, therapeutic dose levels whilst other side-effects are experienced only at higher dose levels. It should be remembered that, in many instances, athletes are taking drugs in doses far in excess of those required for therapeutic purposes and in so doing increase the risk of experiencing side-effects. Side-effects associated with some of the drugs that are commonly misused in sport.

Drug toxicity can to a large extent be predictable. The side-effects of drugs are usually well documented as a result of extensive toxicity studies during the development of the drug and from adverse reaction reporting once the drug is on the market. These predictable toxic effects are more pronounced when the drug is taken in overdose.

This could occur intentionally (suicide, murder) or accidentally. Accidental overdose may result from children mistaking drugs for sweets; iatrogenic (physician produced) toxicity, resulting from incorrect dosing of patients; patient-induced toxicity when the patient does not comply with the prescribed method of treatment. Accidental toxicity can easily occur with athletes who self-medicate themselves without appreciating the full implications of their actions. The naive philosophy that if one tablet produces a particular desired effect then three tablets must be three times as good frequently prevails in these circumstances.

In addition to predictable toxicity, there are numerous ways in which nonpredictable toxicity can occur following the administration of therapeutic or even sub-therapeutic doses of drugs. An example of this is idiosyncrasy where a drug produces an unusual reaction within an individual. This effect is normally genetically determined and is often due to a biochemical deficiency, resulting in the patient's over-reaction to the drug. This may be due to their inability to metabolize the drug.

A second type of non-predictable toxicity is drug allergy. This is an acquired qualitatively altered reaction of the body to a drug. It differs from normal toxicity to drugs in that the patient will only exhibit the reaction if they have been previously exposed to the drug or a closely related chemical. This initial exposure to the drug, or its metabolite, sensitizes the patient by inducing an allergic response. The drug combines with a protein within the body to produce an antigen, which, in turn, leads to the formation of other proteins called antibodies. This reaction in itself does not induce toxic effects. However, subsequent exposure to the drug will initiate an antigen-antibody reaction.

This allergic reaction can manifest itself in a variety of ways. An acute reaction is known as anaphylaxis and normally occurs within one hour of taking the drug. This response frequently involves the respiratory and cardiovascular systems and is often fatal. Subacute allergic reactions usually occur between 1 and 24 hours after the drug is taken and the most common manifestations involve skin reactions, blood dyscrasias, fever and dysfunctions of the respiratory, kidney, liver and cardiovascular systems. Examples of drugs known to produce such allergic responses are aspirin and some antibiotics including penicillins and cephalosporins.

## COMPLEX DRUG REACTIONS

Complex reactions may occur during long-term usage of a drug or where more than one drug is being taken simultaneously.

The dose regime for a drug is chosen with the objective of maintaining a therapeutic dose level within the body. This regime is determined by two factors: the potency of the drug, which indicates the concentration required at each administration and the rate of metabolism and excretion of the drug, which dictates how frequently the dose has to be taken. If the frequency of administration exceeds the elimination rate of a drug, then drug cumulation occurs, thereby increasing the likelihood of toxicity reactions. The reason for a slow elimination may be related to a slow metabolism, a strong tendency to plasma protein binding or an inhibition of excretion such as occurs in patients with kidney disease.

The opposite response to cumulation is seen in patients with drug resistance. This drug resistance may be genetically inherited or acquired. The former type of resistance is not common in humans, though it is an increasing problem in antibacterial therapy where pathogenic microbes can develop genetic changes in their structure or biochemistry which renders them resistant to antibiotic drugs. Acquired resistance to drugs, also known as tolerance, can develop with repeated administration of a drug. Where tolerance occurs, more drug is needed to produce the same pharmacological response.

A very rapidly developing tolerance is known as tachyphylaxis and is seen when a drug is repeatedly administered with a decreasing response to each administration. This is usually caused by a slow rate of detachment of the drug from its receptor sites, so that subsequent doses of the drug are unable to form the drug-receptor complexes which are required to produce an effect. Alternatively the drug may exert its response through the release of an endogenous mediator whose stores become rapidly depleted with consecutive doses of the drug.

There are several instances where the apparent tolerance to drugs cannot be explained in such simple terms and where other factors are evidently involved. A number of drugs acting on the central nervous system, particularly the group known as the narcotic analgesics, produce tolerance which is accompanied by physical dependence. This is a state in which an abrupt termination of the administration of the drug produces a series of unpleasant symptoms known as the abstinence syndrome. These symptoms are rapidly reversed after the readministration of the drug.

A further manifestation of this problem involves psychogenic dependence in which the drug taker experiences an irreversible craving, or compulsion, to take the drug for pleasure or for relief of discomfort. Where more than one drug is being taken there is a possibility for a drug interaction to occur. Less commonly, drugs may interact with certain foodstuffs, particularly milk products in which the calcium can bind to certain drugs and limit their absorption. The interactions are in the main, well documented. Their effects can range from minor toxicity to potential fatality. Such interactions may occur at the site of absorption where one agent may increase or decrease the rate or extent of absorption of the other.

Alternatively drug interactions may affect the distribution metabolism or excretion of the interacting drugs. These types of interaction are known as pharmacokinetic drug interactions. A second type is the pharmacodynamic drug interaction where one drug can affect the response of another drug at its site of action. Interactions involving more than one drug that may be misused in sport.

## DRUGS AND THE LAW

The manufacture and supply of drugs is subject to legal control. This legislation may vary from country to country but the principles are the same.

### The Definition of a Medicinal Product

Medicinal product means any substance which is manufactured, sold, supplied, imported or exported for use in either or both of the following ways:

- Administered to human beings or animals for medicinal purposes
- As an ingredient in the preparation of substances administered to human beings or animals for medicinal purposes

### Classes of Medicinal Products

In the UK, as in many countries, there are three classes of medicinal products:

- General sale list medicines (GSL).
- Pharmacy medicines (P).
- Prescription-only medicines (POM).

The law of the country dictates which medicines may be purchased and which can only be obtained through a prescription. In general these laws are similar from country to country, but exceptions do occur. This may tempt athletes to travel to abroad, specifically to purchase a drug which is more readily available in another country. Alternatively, some drugs may be, illegally, obtained through internet sources.

***Table:*** Drugs present in OTC medicines which are subject to IOC regulations

| Drug | Present in certain medicines for: |
|---|---|
| Ephedrine | Coughs and colds |
| Pseudoephedrine | Hay fever |
| Phenylpropanolamine | |
| Phenylephrine | |
| Morphine | Diarrhoea |
| Caffeine | Pain relief |

Doctors may normally only prescribe drugs or medicines to patients for their licensed therapeutic use. Patients can obtain these prescription-only medicines (POMs) from medical practitioners in a hospital, clinic or community practice. Prescriptions are then dispensed by a pharmacist or, in some cases, by a dispensing doctor. Once the prescription has been dispensed, the medicine becomes the property of the patient. Over-the-counter (OTC) medicines are available for purchase by the general public, without a prescription.

These medicines are normally only available from a pharmacy (P medicines) although some medicines, such as aspirin and other analgesics, may be obtained in small pack sizes from other retail outlets (GSL medicines). OTC drugs pose particular problems for athletes, since a number of drugs subject to IOC regulations are available in OTC preparations. It is the responsibility of the athlete to ensure that they are not taking a banned substance, therefore advice from a pharmacist should be sought when an OTC medicine is purchased. Controlled drugs (CDs), normally those drugs with addictive properties, are subject to further legal restrictions. In most countries CDs include:

- Hallucinogenic drugs (e.g. LSD and marijuana)
- Opiates (narcotic analgesics, e.g. morphine, heroin)
- Amphetamines
- Cocaine

For these drugs, the law states that it is illegal to possess such drugs, except where the user is a registered addict and has obtained their drug legally on prescription.

In some countries anabolic steroids, clenbuterol and some polypeptide hormones are classed as CDs as a further deterrent to their misuse in sport and in body building.

## NUTRITIONAL SUPPLEMENTS

In an attempt to enhance performance through ergogenic aids, without contravening IOC doping control regulations, many athletes have turned to 'natural' products and nutritional supplements. Unlike therapeutic drugs, nutritional supplements are not required to have strong scientific and clinical evidence that they are effective before being allowed to be sold to the public.

They are not subject to the same independent, scientific scrutiny as that for regulated medicines. Manufacturers may therefore make exaggerated claims regarding the ergogenic properties of their products. It is a widely held view by athletes that by using such supplements, performance will be enhanced through replacement of the body's biochemical stores or by modification of the processes involved in weight control and energy function.

Nutritional supplements include vitamins, minerals, carbohydrate, protein and various extracts from plant sources. There is a commonly held view that 'natural' products are, by definition, free of toxic side-effects. This is clearly a misconception, particularly when it is remembered that in the early days of pharmacological science all drugs were derived from plant and animal sources and that many of these derivatives are amongst the most toxic chemicals known to man. Indeed, some nutritional supplements have the potential for harm.

Many of these products are promoted as having ergogenic properties. Such claims are rarely substantiated by sound scientific data in peer-reviewed journals. In recent times, there have been a number of high profile cases involving athletes who have tested positive for the anabolic steroid, nandrolone, where the athlete had claimed that they had ingested the steroid in a 'contaminated' nutritional supplement, an assertion which may be based on truth.

Whether the IOC should revise its doping control regulations, to include nutritional supplements, is debatable.

## Vitamins

Vitamins are frequently taken by athletes on the supposition that they are experiencing a vitamin deficiency due to exercise and training regimes. However, Cotter has suggested that there is little evidence to suggest that exercise would necessitate vitamin supplementation.

In terms of using vitamin supplements as ergogenic aids, the B-complex vitamins have been taken because they are co-enzymes in the processes of red blood cell production and in the metabolism of fats and carbohydrates. Vitamin C is reputed to aid in the wound healing process and vitamin E has been claimed to increase aerobic capacity. All these claims for ergogenic properties of vitamins, in general, there is little evidence available to substantiate these claims. Vitamins, taken in excess, are toxic. This applies particularly to the fatsoluble vitamins (A, D, E and K) which are stored in the body and which can therefore accumulate. Even the water-soluble vitamins (B and C) can produce toxic effects when taken in excess. In general, a balanced diet will provide the necessary nutritional requirements of vitamins. Vitamin supplements are only of benefit where there is a clear deficiency, such as occurs with an exceptional nutritional intake.

## Proteins and Amino Acids

Protein and amino acid supplements are frequently used by athletes, particularly where muscle development is of prime importance. Protein is obviously an essential component of a balanced diet but there is no experimental evidence to show that protein supplementation enhances metabolic activity or leads to increased muscle mass.

Excessive intake of protein can produce toxic effects, due to overproduction of urea with a concomitant loss of water, leading to dehydration with a risk to the competitor of muscle cramp and an impairment of body temperature regulation. Manipulation of diet, to induce metabolic acidosis by reducing carbohydrate intake or increasing fat and protein intake, has shown impaired performance.

The amino acids, arginine and ornithine have been shown to stimulate the release of growth hormone. Such an effect requires intravenous infusion of the amino acids. A similar effect following oral administration of arginine or ornithine has not been established. Furthermore, the literature does not support the idea that growth hormone releasers have an ergogenic effect. In general, it is considered that amino acids do not improve endurance performance and that physically active individuals are advised to obtain necessary amino acids through consumption of natural, high quality protein foods, rather than through supplements.

### Carbohydrate

Sports drinks, used to replace fluid, carbohydrate and electrolytes are widely used by athletes. During endurance exercise, suitable intake of such products has been shown to be beneficial for glycogen-depleted muscles and to enhance performance.

### Ginseng

Ginseng is a herbal preparation comprising a complex mixture of glycosides, known as ginsenosides. There are many varieties of plant from which ginsenosides are extracted and multiple preparations within which they are presented. No two preparations will therefore contain the same combination and dose of ginsenosides. Ginseng has been used for thousands of years, particularly by the Chinese, and many claims have been made as to its therapeutic value. Few scientific experiments have been reported with regard to its performance-enhancing properties failed to find any statistically significant difference in maximum aerobic capacity, heart rate or time to exhaustion during a comparative controlled trial on a small group of marathon runners.

### Creatine

Creatine is an amino acid present in skeletal muscle.

Taking dietary supplements of creatine will add to the whole body creatine pool but the saturation point is soon achieved. Thereafter dietary creatine is simply excreted. Approximately half of the endogenous creatine is in the form of phosphocreatine.

The development of muscle fatigue during exercise is associated with the depletion of muscle phosphocreatine stores. This results in an inability to resynthesize ATP at the normal rate, therefore the force of muscle contraction is reduced. Creatine ingestion will not increase the maximal force or power that an individual can produce, but will improve the ability to maintain performance close to maximum as exercise continues. Parallels to the use of creatine have been drawn with carbohydrate loading.

Creatine has been the subject of many studies, but results are equivocal as to whether it produces ergogenic effects. There are few reliable scientific data on possible adverse effects of creatine but its potential effect on renal dysfunction and electrolyte imbalance, leading to a predisposition to dehydration and heat-related illness, suggests caution in its use.

Creatine is one of the most widely used legal supplements available to athletes, with an estimated 30 to 50 per cent of professional athletes using it on a regular basis.

## L-Carnitine

L-Carnitine is synthesized in the kidneys and liver. It can be obtained through the diet from animal sources. L-Carnitine deficiency is extremely rare. It is required for the transport and oxidation of long-chain fatty acids into mitochondria for the production of energy. It is therefore postulated that ingesting more L-carnitine will lead to more fat being burned to supply energy. Athletes have used its supplementation in the diet to promote fat loss and to enhance aerobic and anaerobic capacity. However, most placebo-controlled trials have failed to demonstrate any improvement in maximal oxygen uptake or in endurance performance in response to oral L-carnitine. A review by Cerretelli and Marconi was unable to show any beneficial effects on performance as a result of L-carnitine supplementation. At the dose ranges used, no reports of toxicity due to L-carnitine were described.

## DRUGS ARE USED IN SPORT

Although there may be many reasons why sportsmen and women use drugs, four main reasons can be identified:

- Legitimate therapeutic use (prescription drug or self-medication).
- Performance continuation (treatment of sports injuries).
- Recreational/social use (legal and illegal).
- Performance enhancement.

In each of the above categories there are drugs which appear in the IOC list of banned substances.

Inevitably, clear distinctions cannot always be made between these uses. It would be easy to say that athletes should avoid taking drugs, for any reason, particularly at the time of a competition. However, there are many circumstances when drug taking is advisable, if not imperative for the general health and well being of the athlete. Therefore it would be prudent for athletes to consider the specific need for taking drugs and the full implications of their action.

There is a heavy reliance upon sophisticated dietary and training programmes to obtain the winning edge. Some so-called vitamin preparations and nutritional supplements may contain banned substances. There is no legal requirement for manufacturers to list all the contents of food supplements. To avoid any in potential conflict with the doping regulations, these supplements are best avoided.

## LEGITIMATE THERAPEUTIC USE OF DRUGS

Like any other person, an athlete is liable to suffer from a major or minor illness that requires treatment with drugs. A typical example might involve a bacterial or fungal infection necessitating the use of an antibiotic or antifungal agent. How many sportsmen or women have experienced athlete's foot? Apart from the slight risk of side-effects due to the drug's action, it is difficult to perceive how such a treatment would affect an athlete's performance. A less common but more serious medical condition would be epilepsy or diabetes. Under these circumstances it would be inconceivable for an athlete to consider participating in sport without regular treatment with drugs. For many minor illnesses, from which we all suffer from time to time, such as coughs, colds, gastrointestinal upsets and hay fever, it is possible to obtain medications without visiting the doctor.

There is a wide range of preparations available for the treatment of minor illnesses which can be purchased from a pharmacy without the need for a doctor's prescription. The drugs contained in these over-the-counter (OTC) medications are relatively less potent than those available on prescription. Athletes should carefully scrutinize the label on any medication or substance which is being taken to ensure that a banned substance is not included in the medicine.

Examples of such substances include the psychomotor stimulant, caffeine and the sympathomimetic amines, ephedrine, pseudoephedrine, phenylpropanolamine and phenylephrine. Though dose levels are low in OTC medications, the sophisticated methods used for the analysis of urine are perfectly capable of detecting these drugs or their metabolites. The IOC introduced urinary cut-off levels for these OTC drugs in the late 1990s. If these drugs are detected in urine samples, at concentrations below the cut-off levels, the athlete will not be sanctioned.

It is also in the athlete's interest, in the event of visiting a medical practitioner, the nature of any drug treatment, to avoid the prescribing of prohibited substances wherever possible. As with any medical condition requiring treatment, a decision needs to be taken as to whether the athlete is fit to compete at all.

### Performance Continuation

Permitted drug treatments to alleviate the symptoms of minor ailments such as sore throats, colds and stomach upsets can be seen as simply allowing the athlete to continue performing during a temporary period of minor ill-health. Athletes frequently experience injuries involving muscles, ligaments and tendons. Provided that the injury is not too serious, it is common for the athlete to take palliative treatment in the form of analgesic and antiinflammatory drugs. This enables the athlete to continue to train and even compete during the period of recovery from the injury. The wisdom of such action is perhaps open to question but the use of analgesics under these circumstances is unlikely to confer an unfair advantage.

The doping regulations restrict the type of analgesics which can be used and control the methods of administration for drugs such as corticosteriods. In weighing up the consequences of giving a pain-killing injection, a doctor would probably take into account: the time available before the athlete is in competition and the extent of the injury. In contrast an athlete is more likely to be thinking about the effort which has been expended in reaching this stage, the remaining opportunities, the rewards from sponsors, the acclaim from family and friends, and often the risks of treatment are inadequately reviewed.

**Table:** Drugs used socially or recreationally that are subject to IOC regulations

| Drug | IOC regulation |
|---|---|
| Amphetamines | Prohibited class IA (stimulants) |
| Cocaine | Prohibited class IA (stimulants) |
| Caffeine | Prohibited class IA (stimulants) (if urine level above 12 μg/ml) |
| Narcotic analgesics | Prohibited class IB (narcotics) |
| Alcohol | Prohibited in certain circumstances, class IIIA |
| Marijuana | Prohibited in certain circumstances, class IIIB |

Certainly, the inappropriate injection of corticosteroids could have deleterious effects on joints systemic complications are not uncommon. Even non-steroidal anti-inflammatory drugs (NSAIDs), such as aspirin, though widely used, are liable to produce adverse effects such as gastrointestinal bleeding and ulceration has suggested that

NSAIDs may not hasten the return of injured athletes back to competition.

### Recreation/social Use

Many cultures, throughout the ages, have used the drugs for social and recreational purposes. These substances range from caffeine, a constituent of beverages frequently consumed in many societies, through the generally socially tolerated drugs, such as alcohol and marijuana, to the hard, addictive drugs such as the narcotic analgesics related to heroin and morphine and the psychomotor stimulants such as cocaine. The use of these drugs, particularly in Western cultures, has grown in recent years. This has been reflected in the increasing numbers of positive test results, particularly for marijuana, from IOC accredited laboratories.

Although these drugs may be taken in a social or recreational setting, they are all potential performance-enhancing drugs, hence their subjection to IOC regulations. Amphetamines, cocaine and narcotic analgesics are banned completely. Caffeine is banned but only if urine concentrations rise above 12 micrograms per millilitre, thus allowing for 'normal' consumption of caffeine-containing beverages. Alcohol and marijuana are prohibited only in certain sports.

### Amphetamines

In the UK, it has been estimated that 10 per cent of 16- to 59-year-olds, rising to 20 per cent of 16- to 29-year-olds have tried amphetamine. Amphetamines are used socially to produce alertness and energy. However, they also impair judgement and concentration and heavy use leads to depression and anxiety. There is a risk of addiction with regular use of amphetamine.

### Cocaine

Cocaine is a powerful stimulant. It is usually inhaled as a powder but a crystalline ('crack') form of cocaine is smoked as a vapour. The complex pharmacology of cocaine leads to a wide spectrum of adverse effects, including a negative effect on glycogenolysis, paranoid psychosis, seizures, hypertension and myocardial toxicity, which could lead to ischaemia, arrhythmias and sudden death, especially following intense exercise. Smoked 'crack' cocaine is more dangerous as the rate of absorption is greater, leading to a more intense effect on the cardiovascular system. After regular use, addictive cravings for cocaine can persist for a period of months.

Some bizarre fatalities have been linked to concomitant use of cocaine with alcohol and anabolic steroids, which may have resulted from the production of a novel, cardiotoxic metabolite, norcocaine.

### Caffeine

Perhaps the most widely used social drug is caffeine, which is present in many of the beverages that we consume daily. These include tea, coffee and many soft drinks. At the levels at which caffeine is normally consumed its pharmacological effects are minimal. However, attempts have been made to use caffeine as a doping agent by taking supplements in the form of tablets or injections. This has necessitated the introduction into the doping control regulations of an upper limit for caffeine present in urine samples (12 micrograms per millilitre).

## NARCOTIC ANALGESICS

The narcotic analgesics are readily absorbed when taken orally, by injection or by inhalation. They are potent drugs whose effects are primarily on the central nervous system. The discovery of opiate receptors within the brain has helped in the understanding of the mode of action of morphine, heroin and other related narcotic analgesics. They appear to be mimicking the effect of certain endogenous opiates, known as endorphins and enkephalin.

They depress certain centres of the brain resulting in reduced powers of concentration, fear and anxiety. Prolonged pain, more so than acute pain, is reduced. Some centres of the brain, such as the vomiting centre and those associated with salivation, sweating and bronchial secretion, are initially stimulated, though they become depressed on continued use of the drugs. The respiratory and cough centres are depressed. Respiration becomes slow, it deepens and may be periodic in nature. Death as a result of overdose of narcotic analgesics normally occurs through respiratory depression. Characteristic side-effects of narcotic analgesics include constricted pupil size, dry mouth, heaviness of the limbs, skin itchiness, suppression of hunger and constipation. Athletes are in danger of addiction to analgesics as they attempt to mask injury to train or to compete.

Narcotic analgesics are renowned for their ability to cause tolerance and dependence in the regular user. Tolerance to the drugs occurs over a period of time and increasing dose levels are needed to produce the same pharmacological effect. Dependence on narcotic analgesics leads to physical withdrawal symptoms.

Symptoms normally begin with sweating, yawning and running of the eyes and nose. These are followed by a period of restlessness which leads to insomnia, nausea, vomiting and diarrhoea. This is accompanied by dilation of the pupils, muscular cramp and a 'goose flesh' feeling of the skin commonly referred to as 'cold turkey'. Relief from the physical withdrawal symptoms of narcotic analgesics can be achieved by the readministration of these drugs, hence the difficulty that addicts experience in trying to terminate their dependence on narcotic analgesics. Methadone, a synthetic opiate, is used to treat heroin addiction. Methadone itself has addictive properties and accounts for many deaths through overdose.

## Alcohol

Alcohol is the most commonly used drug in Britain, with only 7 per cent of males and 13 per cent of females describing themselves as non-drinkers. Though taken for recreational purposes, the effects of alcohol may well be manifested in the field of sport. Some sporting events even take place in an environment where alcohol is freely available both to the spectator and the performer. Alcohol suppresses inhibitions but also impairs judgement and reflexes. Alcoholics risk premature death through cirrhosis of the liver, accidents and suicide.

## Marijuana

Marijuana is a drug derived from the hemp plant and which is normally taken by inhalation in the form of a cigarette but can be taken orally. The precise mode of action of cannabis is not fully understood but the effects produced are principally euphoria and elation accompanied by a loss of perception of time and space. A single 'joint' can slow reactions for up to 24 hours.

Conflicting opinions exist on the dangers associated with prolonged use of cannabis. There is evidence that short-term recall memory can be impaired and that permanent brain damage may be induced. Marijuana can adversely affect psychomotor functions; these effects may last up to 24 hours following its use. Although unlikely to be used as a performance-enhancing substance in sport, events in recent years have shown that marijuana is used as part of the lifestyle of many athletes.

This was illustrated in the landmark case of the Canadian snowboarder, Ross Rebagliati, who tested positive for marijuana and was stripped of his gold medal at the 1998 Winter Olympic Games in Nagano, only to be re-instated when the IOC and the International Ski Federation realized that they were each operating different rules regarding the banning of marijuana. Apart from the validity of the test result, Ross Rebagliati claimed that the marijuana was present in his body through secondary, passive smoking, not as an attempt at performance enhancement.

Controls have been introduced in motorized sports and a number of professional sports such as association football and rugby league have regulated against its use in order to preserve the reputation of the sport and the health of players. The IOC have recently introduced a clause that states that a urine concentration of the metabolite, carboxy-THC, less than 15 nanograms per millilitre, does not constitute doping at Olympic Games.

## PERFORMANCE ENHANCEMENT

This particular area of drug use is potentially the most serious threat to the credibility of competitive sport and has become subject to doping control regulations. It concerns the deliberate, illegitimate use of drugs in an attempt to gain an unfair advantage over fellow competitors. It would be appropriate, at this point, to provide a definition of a performance-enhancing drug. Unfortunately a precise definition is extremely difficult to formulate for a number of reasons.

- A particular drug which may be considered performance enhancing in one sport may well be deleterious to performance in another sport. Drugs with a sedative action, such as alcohol and beta blockers, would be considered useful in events such as rifle shooting where a reduced heart rate and steady stance are important. However, these drugs would be counterproductive, if not dangerous, in most other sports.
- Should performance-enhancing drugs be defined by the fact that they are 'synthetic' or 'unnatural' substances to the body? This type of definition would exclude testosterone and other naturally occurring peptide hormones which are used for illicit purposes. 'Blood doping', the method by which competitors store quantities of their own or other blood in a frozen state and re-infuse it prior to competing in an attempt to increase oxygen carrying capacity, would also be excluded by such a definition.
- Should substances used in special diets, such as vitamin supplements, be classed as performance-enhancing drugs? Certainly other naturally occurring substances, such as creatine and L-carnitine, have been widely used in the expectation that they would enhance performance.
- Perhaps the greatest difficulty in precisely defining performance-enhancing drugs concerns the prescribing and use of drugs which can be perceived

as possessing performance-enhancing properties but which are used for legitimate therapeutic purposes. This problem is readily illustrated when considering athletes who suffer from asthma. One of the most important classes of drugs used for their treatment is the group of bronchodilators, many of which are sympathomimetics and therefore the subject of doping control. Since asthmatic attacks are frequently associated with stress, of which competitive exercise is an extreme case, then this obviously produces severe problems for the asthmatic if they are to avoid transgressing the doping control regulations. Selected bronchodilator sympathomimetics are allowed under doping control regulations.

The issue of performance enhancement is one which will retain media attention at major sporting events. Definitions may actually obscure the fundamental principle as explained by Sir Arthur Porritt, first Chairman of the IOC Medical Commission: 'to define doping is, if not impossible, at best extremely difficult, and yet everyone who takes part in competitive sport or who administers it knows exactly what it means.

The definition lies not in words but in integrity of character'. In essence, it encompasses the principle of cheating, defined in the antidoping regulations of individual sports.

# Chapter 2

# Use and Abuse of Drugs in Sports

## HISTORICAL PERSPECTIVE

The extensive use of medicinal products for the alleviation of the symptoms of disease can be traced back to the Greek physician, Galen, in the third century BC. Interestingly, it was Galen who reported that ancient Greek athletes used stimulants to enhance their physical performance. At the Ancient Olympic Games, athletes had special diets and were reported to have taken various substances to improve their physical capabilities.

The winner of the 200 m sprint at the Olympic Games of 668 BC was said to have used a special diet of dried figs. The Ancient Egyptians used a drink made from the hooves of asses, which had been ground and boiled in oil, then flavoured with rose petals and rose hips, to improve their performance. In Roman times, gladiators used stimulants to maintain energy levels after injury. Similar behaviour by medieval knights has also been noted. In fact throughout history, there are examples that athletes have sought a magic potion to give them that extra edge, to help them take a short cut to achieving a good performance or to enable them to compete under circumstances when otherwise it might not have been possible, such as injury or illness. Today's athletes may simpiy be following previous traditions.

The use of drugs is not restricted to humans, horses were also found to have been doped. The intention was not always to improve performance, it may have been to 'nobble' the opposition. Doping of horses was prohibited in 1903, however it was not until saliva testing was used effectively in 1910 that horse doping could be proven. Subsequent improvements in technology to identify the vast range of substances prohibited in equestrian sports has led to blood and urine testing being carried out regularly at race meetings and more recently at no notice at stables.

In the nineteenth century, swimmers in the Amsterdam canal races were thought to have used some form of stimulant, as were cyclists in the endurance events. Caffeine, cocaine, strychnine, ether, alcohol and oxygen were reported to have been used alone and in combination. Probably the first reported drug-related death in sport was the cyclist Arthur Linton in 1896, who was reportedly administered strychnine by his coach.

Although later reports suggest that Linton died of typhoid fever, his coach had been banned from the sport, presumably for his part in doping. Another British athlete, Thomas Hicks came close to death after winning the 1904 Olympic Marathon in St Louis USA, following the use of strychnine and brandy. His life was probably saved by the actions of doctors at the finish.

Up to the middle of the nineteenth century, there was little documentary evidence available to substantiate the hypothesis that drugs had been used in sport. Whilst there were no control mechanisms in place in sport, the Dangerous Drugs Act was introduced in 1920 to restrict the availability of cocaine and opium by prescription only. Perhaps the dearth of evidence for the abuse of drugs in sport up to the Second World War is reflective of the paucity of substances available, coupled with their low potency, when compared with the powerful chemicals of today.

Around the time of the Second World War, the development of amphetamine-like substances reached a peak. These drugs were administered to combat troops in order to enhance their mental awareness and to delay the onset of fatigue. Not surprisingly, in the 1940s and 1950s, amphetamines became the drugs of choice for athletes, particularly in sports such as cycling, where the stimulant effects were perceived to be beneficial to enhancing sporting performance in sprint and stamina events.

Deaths of sportsmen from amphetamine abuse in the 1960s demonstrated how widespread drug abuse had become. At the 1960 Rome Olympics, the cyclist Knud Jensen died on the opening day of the Games as he competed in the 100 km team time trial. Two team mates were also taken to hospital. The post-mortem revealed traces of amphetamine and nicotinyl nitrate in Jensen's blood. In 1967, the death of the British cyclist Tommy Simpson during the Tour de France was televised across the world.

Weeks later, it was revealed that traces of amphetamine, methylamphetamine and cognac were found in Simpson's body. Amphetamine was also found in the pocket of his jersey and his luggage. Two other deaths in cycling and football were recorded in the next year. Further evidence of the increase in amphetamine abuse came from the admission by the British athlete Alan Simpson that he has used them during the 1966 Commonwealth Games.

The phenomenon of drug use in sport must be seen in parallel with two other factors. First, the sixties heralded a more liberal approach to experimentation in drug taking, particularly among the followers of pop music. Second and of far greater significance, a 'pharmacological revolution' began in the 1960s. The search by pharmaceutical companies for more potent, more selective and less toxic drugs resulted in a vast array of powerful agents capable of altering many biochemical, physiological and psychological functions in the body. Not surprisingly some athletes saw, in these

chemical agents, a means of enhancing performance beyond anything that they could achieve by hard work and rigorous training. Moreover, it offered a greater menu of choice for athletes to use. Athletes could simply select the most specific drugs to meet their particular needs for improving performance.

Originally athletes used amphetamines and other stimulants, mainly on the day of, or during, performance. There was growing evidence that these drugs might be linked with sudden collapse or death, usually from cardiac or respiratory arrest, particularly during competition, yet the long term side-effects on the body were regarded as minor. By comparison the drugs which emerged in the 1950s among body builders in America and later among athletes and weightlifters, the anabolic steroids, were a different story. These drugs, whilst increasing size and strength in some athletes, also cause significant side-effects.

The advantage these drugs offered was their usefulness to an athlete in training, in preparation for a competition. This was especially important in the early days of testing programmes to control the use of drugs. The desire to enhance performance for national prestige and ideological supremacy dominated the sporting world in the 1970s and 1980s. The Stasi files documented the governmentally organized steroid doping of the German Democratic Republic ; it is possible that other programmes may not have been as well documented or evident.

Drug misuse today has increased in sophistication, athletes are seeking out ways to improve performance using the most advanced technology. The former coach to Ben Johnson, Charlie Francis wrote There are thousands of possible synthetic permutations of the testosterone molecule. The great majority of these steroids remain an unexplored frontier...private laboratories stand ready to synthesise any number of these steroids-and keep the athletes ahead of the game'.

Unfortunately, evidence for the performance-enhancing properties of drugs is sparse. It has not been possible to undertake controlled trials, where drugs could be evaluated on large groups of individuals and compared with a placebo, preferably on a double-blind basis where neither the tester nor the individuals being tested are aware of whether they are taking the drug or the placebo.

This approach would have been similar to that adopted by drug companies in order to establish whether new drugs are effective therapeutic agents. Clearly there are logistical and ethical reasons why such trials could not take place.

Consequently, much of the rationale behind drug taking in sport is based on hypothetical performance-enhancing properties, speculation, misinformation from 'underground' booklets and sheer ignorance. In addition, little cognizance is taken of the side-effects associated with drugs and the potential adverse effect these may have on performance. Statistics published by the IOC accredited laboratories since 1993 indicate anabolic steroids are the most frequently detected substance, consistently representing a significant percentage of the total findings.

## DEFINITION OF DOPING

The origin of the word doping is interesting, dop referred to a stimulant drink used in tribal ceremonies in South Africa around the eighteenth century. Dop first appeared in an English dictionary in 1889, it was described as a narcotic potion for racehorses to reduce their performance. Contemporary use has extended the definition to include the improvement of performance. As practice has developed, the definition also refers to maintenance of performance and manipulation of the testing procedures by the use of doping classes or methods.

So the word 'doping' is now used to describe not only the misuse of drugs by sportsmen and women, but also the use of other methods of improving performance or of attempting to manipulate the test. This definition is not without controversy. There are many different ways athletes attempt to improve their performance, for example, altitude training, diet, biomechanical analysis and psychological preparation. However, these techniques are generally accepted as a part of an athlete's training and preparation regime.

The doping definition of the IOC is based on the banning of pharmacological classes. Rule 29A of the Olympic Charter states: 'Doping is forbidden. The IOC Medical Commission shall prepare a list of prohibited classes of drugs and of banned procedures.' Further explanation of this approach is given in the introductory paragraph to the published list. The definition has the advantage that also new drugs, some of which may be especially designed for doping purposes, are banned'.

This definition demonstrates the concern for the increasing sophistication in chemical technology, as athletes and their scientists seek chemical agents to improve performance but which may not yet be covered by current regulations, a veritable competition between the testing regime and some athletes.

A comparison of initial attempts to define doping illustrates the difficulties of reflecting practice in words. An early definition from the International Amateur Athletic Federation (IAAF) referred to: The administration of, or use by a competing athlete of any substance foreign to the body or any physiological substance taken in abnormal quantity or taken by an abnormal route of entry into the body with the sole intention of increasing in an artificial and unfair manner his/her performance in competition. When necessity demands medical treatment with any substance which, because of its nature, dosage, or application is able to boost the athlete's performance in competition in an artificial and unfair manner, this too is regarded as doping.

This definition could be challenged on many points; not all substances are foreign to the body, the issue of intention and the link with performance improvement.

Legal challenges have encouraged the progress of a definition of doping and most sports federations have adopted an absolute offence approach. The more recent definition of the IAAF states:

Doping is strictly forbidden and is an offence under IAAF rules. An offence of doping takes place when either

- A prohibited substance is found to be present within an athlete's body tissue or fluids; or
- An athlete takes advantage of a prohibited technique; or
- An athlete admits having used or taken advantage of a prohibited substance or prohibited technique.

Further explanations refer to metabolites of a prohibited substance and to a more detailed definition of prohibited techniques, including blood doping and use of substances to alter the integrity and validity of urine samples used in doping control. Ancillary offences such as failure or refusal to submit to doping control are indicated, as are assisting or inciting others to use a prohibited substance or technique.

Already the definition has been extended, not only to take account of a move from the analysis of urine to blood or other body tissues, but also to supporting evidence of doping, admission, supply and not submitting to a test. The British Athletic Federation originally tackled the issue of availability for testing by including a regulation about notification of address, if an athlete is absent from the home address for a period of 5 days or longer. This in itself may be regarded as a doping offence, and whilst it seems far removed from the misuse of drugs, it is further evidence of the need to reflect practice in the rules and procedures that control doping in sport. More recently the International Amateur Athletic Federation has reduced the period of absence requiring notification to 3 days.

One of the problems with a definition based upon a list of substances is that not all sports may adopt the same classification. The offence of doping may vary between sports. This situation occurred during the 1988 Tour de France, when the Spanish cyclist Pedro Delgardo tested positive for a substance banned by the IOC. However, because this substance was not banned by the International Cycling Union, no penalty could be imposed.

A similar situation arose at the 1998 Nagano Winter Olympics when the Canadian snow boarder Ross Rebagliati tested positive for marijuana. The true construction of the IOC Rules regarded marijuana as a doping offence, however the absence of an agreement between the IOC and the relevant international sports federation about the status of this substance led the Court of Arbitration for Sport to rule that no specific prohibition had been made.

The majority of sports have adopted the list of prohibited classes published by the IOC and more recently taken over by the World Anti-Doping Agency. Differences still exist between the IOC list and the prohibited substances list of some international federations. Whilst the opportunity to create a more sports-specific list would make the testing more relevant, it might also presuppose a link between performance enhancement and the prohibited substances. The most recent definition comes from the Olympic Movement Anti-Doping Code of 1999, which defines doping as

- The use of an expedient (substance or method) which is potentially harmful to athletes' health and/or capable of enhancing their performance; or
- The presence in the athlete's body of a prohibited substance or evidence of the use thereof or evidence of the use of a prohibited method.

This definition sets out clearly the basis for defining doping as a strict liability offence; it is the very presence of a prohibited substance that triggers the disciplinary process. Despite this, there have still been a number of challenges about the performance-enhancing effects of substances detected or the absence of any health consequences for the detection of a substance.

Defining doping as the use of prohibited substances places great emphasis on the role of a drug testing programme to detect banned substances. Not all banned substances are detectable. Legal challenges have led to more specific explanations within the regulations, including the presence of metabolites, the use of substances to alter the validity or integrity of the urine sample, refusal or failure to submit to doping control, and assisting or inciting others to use a prohibited substance or technique. This extension of the definition of doping to beyond the scientific evidence of substance misuse creates an even greater challenge of bringing sufficient proof.

## A REVIEW OF THE IOC LIST OF DOPING CLASSES AND METHODS

### Doping Classes

Since the IOC list of doping classes was first published in 1967, it has evolved gradually to its present form. Five doping classes are now recognized by the IOC, although in 1992 the list had grown to six classes. The first IOC list included stimulants and narcotic analgesics. Anabolic steroids were first banned in 1974 by the IOC Medical Commission when the technology to detect these substances became available and in response to the concern about potential abuse during training. Although the addition of anabolic steroids to the list recognized their potential for abuse by athletes, testing was based at competitions, so the regime of drug use was not effectively addressed. The introduction of out of competition testing acknowledged the need to control substances both in and out of competition.

A detection method for testosterone was introduced at the 1982 Commonwealth Games in Brisbane. The inclusion of this substance in the IOC list in 1983 was significant as it was the first endogenous or naturally produced steroid to be banned. Up to that time banned substances were foreign to the body. Scientists were faced with the problem of determining limits for the concentration of a natural substance in the body, beyond which it could be determined doping had taken place.

Detection of testosterone (T) was based upon a comparison of hormones in the body, luteinizing hormone (LH) secreted by the pituitary gland and epitestosterone (E) secreted by the testes. Originally the ratio for testosterone to epitestosterone (T/E) determination was set at 6:1, however in 1992 the IOC introduced evaluation criteria for T/E ratios above 6 and below 10. If the ratio exceeded 6 to 1, further investigations were recommended, including a review of previous tests, endocrinological investigations and longitudinal testing over several months.

A doping offence would be reported, unless it could be determined that the ratio was due to a physiological or pathological condition. A ratio that exceeded 10 would be regarded as a doping offence. Challenges to the acceptability of the IOC specified level have criticized the arbitrary nature of the reporting level set by the IOC, especially as it is an endogenous substance. Confusion about responsibility and precise requirements for an independent medical examination to determine whether a medical condition is responsible for the unusual ratio have caused difficulty in cases where the governing body has been primarily for determining whether a doping offence has occurred.

A quantitative test for the stimulant, caffeine was introduced at the Olympic Games in Sarajevo and Los Angeles in 1984. The concentration level was originally set at 15 micrograms per millilitre (μg/ml). This was reduced to 12 μg/ml in 1988.

In 1985, the IOC added the classes of beta blockers and diuretics to the list. For the first time, the IOC acknowledged the need for greater sports specificity in the application of the doping classes. Supporting information for the class of beta blockers referred to the 'misuse of beta blockers in some sports where physical activity is of no or little importance'. This was unlikely to include endurance events.

Some International Federations have adopted the IOC's list but have also taken an opportunity to apply the doping classes more specifically to their sport and set aside the inclusion of all the doping classes. Thus not all sports have included beta blockers and/ or diuretics in their regulations. In 1993, the IOC moved beta blockers of doping classes to the 'Classes of drugs subject to certain restrictions', indicating that they should be tested for only in those sports where they are likely to enhance performance.

Probenecid and other masking agents were added in 1987, together with human chorionic gonadotrophin (hCG). Growth hormone (GH) and other peptide hormones were included in the 1989 list under the new class of peptide hormones. This class also includes corticotrophin (ACTH) and erythropoietin (EPO). The development of recombinant technology has increased the availability of GH in synthetic form. The evolution of the list is clearly indicative of the increasing sophistication of techniques to improve performance and a growing concern to regulate in the absence of unequivocal detection methods.

The classifications have also been broadened by the term 'and related compounds' to the list of examples of each class. Through this route the precursors of nandrolone were captured through tests as a metabolite of the anabolic steroid nandrolone.

## Doping Methods

Blood doping was banned in 1985 although no detection method existed at that time. Its inclusion came about as a result of admissions of blood doping from long distance runners and latterly from members of the US cycling team. Evidence emerged that US cyclists had received blood transfusions two days prior to the start of the Los Angeles Olympics. A detection method was not available, so early offences of blood doping rested on admissions from athletes. Only recently has the testing procedure in some sports been extended to allow for the collection of blood samples. Urine samples are also collected from athletes. The first blood testing was carried out at the 1988 World Ski Championship and continued in a limited way in skiing and track and field athletics. Blood testing at the Olympic Games was first carried out during the Winter Olympic Games in Lillehammer in 1994.

The samples are investigated for evidence of homologous blood cells, i.e. blood other than the athlete's own. Current scientific knowledge is insufficient to confirm the use of autologous (same) blood, although scientists have made advances in detecting refrigerator-stored blood. Most recent advances in blood testing techniques have focused upon erythropoeitin and other plasma expanders. This has involved the testing of blood parameters, haemoglobin, haematocrit and reticulocytes. Athletes failing to achieve the required parameters from the blood sample provide a urine sample for more detailed analysis for the presence of blood doping.

Pharmacological, chemical and physical manipulation was also added to the list in 1985 in an attempt to control the growing trend of deception that had entered into the procedure. Anecdotal evidence of urine substitution, catheterization and in some cases actually having the sample provided by impostors threatened the effectiveness of the testing system. Athletes also tried to use substances to inhibit renal excretion, such as probenecid and to titrate testosterone/

epitestosterone levels in the body. Where evidence of these manipulation techniques emerged the classification of doping methods enabled the sports authorities to act. Significantly, very few cases of manipulation are ever confirmed as doping offences, indicating perhaps the difficulty of presenting evidence.

The most well-known case to have been heard was that involving Katrin Krabbe, Silke Muller and Grit Breuer, whose urine samples provided during a training session in South Africa bore such a similarity it led to the allegation that they had been provided by the same person. Evidence brought forward at the disciplinary hearing in London in June 1992 concluded that the same individual probably had provided the samples and that an opportunity had existed for the athletes to catheterize urine from another person prior to the sample collection. The offences could not be pursued as the doping regulations of the German Athletic Federation (DLV) did not provide the authority to collect samples out of competition abroad.

## CLASSES OF DRUGS SUBJECT TO CERTAIN RESTRICTIONS

In addition to the doping classes and methods noted above, there are restrictions on specific pharmacological classes in certain sports. The responsibility is with the international federation to determine whether controls on these substances are necessary. Within this group, alcohol and marijuana are prohibited. Alcohol may be tested for by breath or blood testing; actual levels may vary between sports that restrict the use of alcohol. Control of the abuse of alcohol has taken on a different dimension with the timing of breath testing prior to a competition in order that offenders may be withdrawn.

Injectable local anaesthetics and corticosteroids are permitted under restricted conditions and only if medically justified. No published limit has been set for the use of these substances and it is likely that abuse continues. Sport has now inherited a substantial list of prohibited substances that reflects, in part, the practices of athletes, but also the concerns of pharmacologists that loopholes might exist in the regulations that would allow athletes to design their own doping substances. Whilst the IOC was the originator of a general list for sports (that has been welcomed with different degrees of acceptance by some sports), the World Anti-Doping Agency has taken on the task of developing a list that can be generally applied and yet has sport's specificity. The World Anti-Doping Code is expected to be published by the 2004 Olympic Games in Athens.

There is considerable debate among the medical profession and sporting fraternity as to whether some of the drugs should remain on the list. Much will depend upon the agreed definition of doping. However, the justification for inclusion of substances is not simply based on their potential for performance enhancement. Unfortunately, the list of doping classes has also become a reference point for those considering using drugs to improve performance, without any real understanding of why they are prohibited or what their effects are.

The mere presence of one of the banned drugs, or their metabolites, in a urine sample collected as part of an authorized testing programme may constitute an offence. In the case of caffeine and testosterone, a quantitative analysis of the urine is required. This will determine whether the drug is present in the urine in quantities significantly greater than those 'normally' found in urine.

Initially, the IOC list only included drugs for which a specific, conclusive testing procedure was available. However, in recent years blood doping and peptide hormones have been included, for which confirmatory tests were unavailable. Research into definitive detection methods is on-going and likely to catch athletes unaware.

The use of blood rather than urine sampling would significantly assist testing of these substances; however, there are ethical, legal, procedural and medical issues to be resolved before this form of testing becomes more widely accepted and useful. 'Blood sampling is less meaningful when performed after a competition; blood sampling should be performed before competition and in the training periods'. This hypothesis continues to have a major impact upon the perceived effectiveness of blood testing.

Changing trends in the misuse of drugs in sport have been reflected in the periodic revision of the list of doping classes and methods. Unfortunately the absence of a strict timetable for this revision has led to confusion in the past, the danger is this can cause some delay in the implementation of revised regulations or the rapid introduction of regulations without warning. In anticipation of potential challenges to the testing programmes, particularly at major games, sports organizations are beginning to establish their own timetables.

For example the Commonwealth Games Federation, for the Manchester 2002 Games, operated from the list of doping classes which had been in place three months before the Games began. This was to stop late additions, particularly those involving therapeutic medications, catching athletes unaware. The World Anti-Doping Agency has clarified the timetable for revising and publicizing the list. In future an annual revision and specified introduction date will assist the sporting world in understanding its own rules.

For each of the classes of drugs, the prohibited substances classes are supported by lists of examples of the drugs that fall within that group. The lists are not comprehensive and include the phrase 'and related substances'. The term describes drugs that are related to that class by their pharmacological actions and/or chemical structure. This explanation was added to the 1993 IOC list. The principal reason for giving such a broad definition is to ensure that any new drug which is introduced on to the market and which belongs to a prohibited class is automatically included in the list.

This avoids the need for a continual update of the lists and prevents an athlete from claiming the substance they have taken is not covered by the regulations. The drugs are listed under their generic name, which identifies the particular chemical substance(s) the drug contains. However, the same drug may be manufactured and sold by several different drug companies throughout the world and each company will use their own commercial name to describe that drug; for example, the analgesic paracetamol (generic name) can be bought under the commercial names Panadol, Disprol, Paldesic and Calpol. Paracetamol is permitted under current doping regulations.

The situation is further complicated where, as frequently occurs, a drug is combined with other drugs within a medication. This commonly occurs with the sympathomimetics combined with other substances in cough remedies and there are many examples of where the second substance is prohibited. Paracetamol is often combined with caffeine and codeine, although the latter is now permitted for therapeutic use.

## THE RATIONALE FOR DRUG MISUSE IN SPORT

As the motivation for drug misuse cannot be determined from the analysis of the urine sample, it requires further investigation with the athlete and of their environment. The opportunity to do this is not provided for within the rules of many sports federations. Investigations into the environment in which doping has taken place have primarily been led by governments or the judiciary, rarely has sport been able to undertake the thorough investigations required. The introduction of an independent observer system under the World Anti-Doping Agency and certified quality systems helps to normalize external monitoring, investigation and reporting.

Have we...lost track of what athletic competition is about? Is there to much emphasis by the public and by the media on the winning of a gold medal in Olympic competition as the only achievement worthy of recognition? The substances that have been prohibited or restricted for sportsmen and women are only a minority of the number of drugs and medications available. The reasons why they may be misused by athletes are many and various, however the justification for controlling the use of drugs is simply explained: 'the use of doping agents in sport is both unhealthy and contrary to the ethics of sport'.

There may be many reasons why an athlete uses drugs in sport. If the motivation is performance enhancement, the type of drug used will depend on its pharmacological action and the sporting activity the athlete is involved in. To understand why athletes may use prohibited or restricted substances, the effects and perceived benefits to athletes of doping substances. However, there are athletes who combine substances in an attempt to increase their effects or to counter side-effects.

## Stimulants

By comparison with other classes of drugs, stimulants have probably been misused in sport over the longest period of time. Their main purpose has been to improve performance by the general action of stimulation of the central nervous system. Athletes may use stimulants to reduce tiredness, or to increase alertness, competitiveness and aggression. They are considered to have a performance-enhancing effect on endurance events as well as on explosive power activities because of an increased capacity to exercise strenuously and a reduction in sensitivity to pain.

Probably one of the earliest reasons for the use of stimulants was to help athletes through 'the pain barrier'. Stimulants are more likely to be used on the day of a competition; however, it seems likely that athletes now consider the use of stimulants in training to allow the intensity of the training session to be increased. There is, however, little scientific evidence available to suggest that stimulants do improve performance. As stimulants could increase an athlete's aggression towards other competitors or officials, there are potential dangers involved in their misuse in contact sports.

The stimulant class includes psychomotor stimulants, sympathomimetics and miscellaneous CNS stimulants. Examples of this class include caffeine, the amphetamines, ephedrine and cocaine.

Caffeine is the pharmacologically active substance which occurs in social drinks such as tea, coffee and cola. The amount which normally occurs varies according to the type of drink and the way it has been prepared. Relatively high doses are needed to reduce fatigue and the side-effects of tremor may be detrimental. According to one study, doses of about 1000 mg would be needed to produce caffeine levels exceeding 12 μg/ml in the urine, the current quantitative level set by the

IOC. Concentrations found in tea and coffee are, on average, 50-80 mg and 80-150 mg, respectively. In addition, caffeine is a constituent of some medications such as cold preparations and migraine treatment, usually in quantities of less than 100 mg per dose. Caffeine produces a mild central stimulation, similar to amphetamine, reducing fatigue, increasing concentration and arousal. Physiological effects include increased heart rate and output, increased metabolic rate and urine production. High doses can cause anxiety, insomnia and nervousness.

Amphetamines are a controlled drug under the UK Misuse of Drugs Act 1971. Although they have been prescribed as appetite suppressants and for the treatment of narcolepsy, amphetamines are known to produce dependence, often in increasing doses. Athletes have probably used amphetamines to sharpen reflexes, reduce tiredness and increase euphoria. However, competitors have also died as a result of amphetamine misuse, as they raise blood pressure which, with increased physical activity and peripheral vasoconstriction, makes it difficult for the body to cool down. If the body overheats and is unable to cool down, it dehydrates and blood circulation decreases. The heart and other organs are unable to work normally.

The sympathomimetic drug, ephedrine, has been used in cold treatments and originally in bronchodilation for asthmatics. However, it is now regarded as less suitable for use as a bronchodilator having been linked with cardiac arrhythmias. Ephedrine is likely to be misused for its euphoric effect, but could also be used inadvertently as an over-the-counter medication to treat cold or influenza symptoms. Because of the possibility that inadvertent use could be argued, it is likely that athletes would try to misuse ephedrine to obtain an amphetamine-like euphoria.

Cocaine has been used in a variety of treatments for many years; it even appeared as an original ingredient in Coca-Cola until it was removed in 1903. Its therapeutic indication is as a local anaesthetic, though it is likely to be misused for its euphoric effects and feeling of decreased fatigue. Moreover it has the potential for use as a recreational drug arising from the lifestyle some athletes engage in. Cocaine has been directly linked to the deaths of US basketball player Len Bias and American Footballer Don Rogers. In sprint-trained athletes, cocaine is likely to increase heat and lactic acid formation, which coupled with the vasoconstriction effect contributes to fatal cardiac damage.

One of the more controversial groups of stimulants are the β2 -agonists, which are frequently used in medicine as an anti-asthmatic treatment. Up to 1993, the IOC permitted the following β2 -agonists by inhalation only: bitolterol, orciprenaline, rimiterol, salbutamol, terbutaline.

In 1993, this group was reduced to two β2 -agonists, salbutamol and terbutaline, it currently includes formoterol and salmeterol in addition to these two. Concerns about the potential mild anabolic effects, and misuse of β2 -agonists by inhalation, have led to a tightening of the regulations. The IOC have created a special section for this particular group of drugs under the class of anabolic agents.

Sports are also beginning to regulate potential misuse of asthma inhalers in a different and more applicable way. Rumours circulated that use of asthma inhalers just prior to competing would improve performance. This appeared to have gained credence among competitive swimmers who believed that use of an inhaler would enable them to take in more air before diving into the water, to stay underwater for longer and therefore to experience less resistance. Reduction of resistance might provide the split second advantage needed to win. To counter this, the governing body has ruled that an athlete must move away from the pool-side to receive treatment and to allow time for recovery. Similar action is being considered by other sports.

## Narcotic Analgesics

Pain relief was one of the earliest medical uses of drugs. Narcotic analgesics act on the brain to reduce the amount of pain felt from injury or illness. In sports, the use of powerful pain-killing drugs might enable an athlete to exert themselves beyond their normal pain threshold. There are considerable dangers in this to the health of the individual athlete, who may try to compete or train despite an existing serious injury which could lead to further injury, permanent damage or to physical dependence on the drugs themselves.

Narcotic analgesics have strong addictive properties and, as such, are tightly controlled by legislation in most countries. The IOC regulations apply specifically to the opiate analgesics including derivatives such as morphine, heroin, pethidine and dextropropoxyphene. Particular mention is made in the IOC regulations of those substances which are permitted, dextromethorphan, pholcodeine and diphenoxylate. One of the milder forms, codeine, was previously prohibited for use. Codeine is widely available in a variety of medicines, analgesics, diarrhoea suppressants, cough mixtures and cold remedies, over-the-counter.

The level of codeine present in these medicines is too low to induce the serious adverse effects associated with narcotic analgesics but its availability may have caused difficulties in self-medication without contravening doping regulations. In 1993, the IOC removed codeine from the list of examples of prohibited substances and initially indicated that it was now permitted for therapeutic use. (A revised version of the IOC list which appeared later in the year did not contain this advice.) Whilst this move is likely to be welcomed by athletes, it does, however, cause difficulties for testing, since codeine is metabolized to morphine, among other substances, in the body. Not all sports federations had agreed with the IOC's previous ruling prohibiting codeine; track and field athletics, for example, had permitted the therapeutic use of codeine. In terms of treatments for pain, nonsteroidal anti-inflammatory drugs, such as aspirin, remain permitted.

## Anabolic Agents

In March 1993, the IOC changed its classification of anabolic steroids to anabolic agents and created two subgroups: androgenic anabolic steroids and other anabolic agents and β2- agonists (e.g. clenbuterol). This realignment of anabolic agents within a broader group was a further clarification of the IOC's position in respect of clenbuterol. Apparent confusion about its status may have led to use by athletes and body builders for performance enhancement reasons. In particular, a rather acrimonious and lengthy debate followed reports of clenbuterol use by athletes prior to the 1992 Barcelona Olympics and the classification of clenbuterol as an anabolic agent as well as a stimulant.

The reports, having arisen from out-of-competition testing which concentrates primarily upon anabolic agents, masking agents and peptide hormones, have been challenged by the athletes concerned and the matter remains unresolved. Clenbuterol has been shown in animal studies to increase skeletal muscle mass and reduce body fat.

The trend away from the relatively short term use of stimulants towards longer term administration of androgenic anabolic steroids (AAS) aimed at increasing performance by modifying muscle size or nature marks a serious departure into planned and organized drug misuse. The steroid drugs currently in use are largely chemically derived alternatives to naturally occurring testosterone. Contrary to popular belief, oral administration of androgenic anabolic steroids is more dangerous than injection of these drugs.

Oral forms have to be broken down in the liver first, creating risks of liver disease; injectable forms are oil based and fat soluble making their release into the body system slower, as fat stores are broken down. Orally active AAS are water soluble and are likely to have a shorter clearance time in the body, making their use more popular among athletes subject to drug testing. However, clearance times are also likely to be dose related and are difficult to calculate with any certainty. The use of androgenic anabolic steroids by athletes from certain sports has become widespread in particular in strength, power, body-building and stamina activities. Whilst the pretext for using AAS is to increase muscle development, there is no strong evidence to show that AAS exert a direct growth-promoting effect on muscles. The exception here would be in female athletes and pre-pubescent males.

Attempts to interfere with the ageing process have been made since the first use of 'monkey glands' 100 years ago. Emphasis has mainly been on the male sex hormones, such as testosterone, and their ability to improve the quality of life. The protein-building properties of anabolic steroids had led to the hope that they might be more widely useful in medicine, but this has not been realized due to the adverse side-effects reported. The side-effects associated with androgenic anabolic steroids are extremely serious, particularly the consequences of long-term or high dosage.

Regrettably these side-effects do not seem to have deterred athletes, in particular body builders, from misusing steroids (and other drugs to counter some of the side-effects). The following summarizes some of the main reasons why athletes would use androgenic anabolic steroids and why there are concerns about their use.

The side-effects associated with these drugs are extremely serious, particularly the consequences of their long-term use. Dr Robert Voy warned 'there is absolutely no anabolic-androgenic steroid that affects an athlete anabolically without also affecting him or her androgenically... There isn't an anabolic-androgenic steroid an athlete can take to increase muscle mass, endurance, or speed without risking dangerous hormonal side-effects.'

To overcome the difficulties of administering testosterone orally, the chemically derived versions attempted to separate the androgenic properties (masculinization in females, acne, suppression of testicular function) from the anabolic effects of increased muscle mass and body weight, positive nitrogen balance and the general feeling of well being. This separation has not proved possible, so athletes who wish to use these drugs have to accept the androgenic and anabolic effects.

Use of steroid drugs alone will not improve performance. An athlete would require a high protein intake and intensive training if gains in performance are to be achieved. Research suggests that physical performance is enhanced in a limited way, for example as increased strength but not endurance. However, another effect of androgens in the body is to stimulate the production of endogenous erythropoietin, which would lead to an increase in the number and stability of red blood cells.

It is in the two groups of individuals who are most likely to derive benefit from muscular development that the greatest risk of toxic side-effects occurs. Females will undergo masculinization resulting in hair growth on the face and body, irreversible voice changes and serious disturbances to the menstrual cycle. Adolescent males may experience stunting of growth. All users are likely to experience severe acne on the face and body. In males, depending on the types and doses, the side-effects may include gynaecomastia, heart disease, hypertension, liver toxicity and premature baldness.

Users seem likely to ignore these side-effects, particularly as they may not be obviously apparent. The side-effects which are more serious and potentially fatal are side-effects such as atherosclerosis and fluid retention, both of which may lead to cardiovascular problems, and the increased risk of developing cancer of the liver and kidney.

Another important point to remember is that some reported adverse side-effects may coincide with other factors. Body builders, for example, use a wide variety of other drugs to achieve their body image, such as diuretics, insulin, thyroid hormone and growth hormone in addition to steroids. They also ingest many nutritional supplements and sports supplements which are unregulated and may contain contraindicated substances. suggests that some of the effects (e.g. thrombotic stroke) may be uniquely related to the extraordinary doses used by athletes. In fact, he indicates that for some the only limit seems to be cost and availability of the drugs.

Unfortunately the reputation of anabolic steroids as performance-enhancing drugs has achieved a considerable level of notoriety among athletes, whilst the adverse effects, being more long term, have been ignored. It is debatable whether an extensive programme of education and information to warn athletes of the consequences of androgenic anabolic steroid use in a non-therapeutic manner would bring about a change in behaviour and attitude. Angela Issajenko, Olympic silver medallist, confessed to taking anabolic steroids, hCG and testosterone.

I came to the conclusion that people I'd compete with in Moscow were also on anabolics so I decided that was the way to go. People are not concerned with the side-effects, or so called side-effects, with anabolic use. They don't believe it. First and foremost what comes to mind is this is going to help me be the best in the world. Whatever comes later, comes later.

Charlie Francis, Ben Johnson's former coach, speaking at the Dubin Inquiry stated 'It's pretty clear that steroids are worth the price of a metre at the highest levels of sport'.

The introduction of an out-of-competition testing programme has added a potential deterrent to steroid use for those subject to a testing programme; however, the programme is not implemented on any large scale world-wide and certainly lacks the necessary co-ordination.

**Diuretics**

Diuretics have the pharmacological effect of elimination of fluid from the body. As such they have a medical use in removing excess fluid due to heart failure, and in lower doses to reduce blood pressure. These drugs may, however, be misused by sportsmen and women for three main reasons. First, they may be taken to effect acute reduction of weight to meet weight-class limits. In this respect they may offer a potential advantage in sports such as boxing, judo or weightlifting where competition is in weight categories. Second, diuretics may be used to overcome fluid retention induced by androgenic anabolic steroids.

This could be useful to body builders trying to obtain a 'cut' look. Third, athletes may use diuretics to modify the excretion rate of urine and to alter urinary concentrations of prohibited drugs. An athlete likely to be selected for drug testing might attempt to increase the volume of urine and to dilute the doping agent, or its metabolites in the urine. The sophistication of detection techniques means that this form of manipulation is unlikely to be effective.

Diuretics are controlled in competition because of their weight reduction potential. Out of competition there is careful monitoring of their use as a manipulation technique. Before, during and after exercise, athletes should take in considerable amounts of fluid. Competitors who misuse diuretics could suffer from dehydration; insufficient fluid in the body may cause faintness, muscle cramps, headaches and nausea. Losing too much water could also cause the kidneys and heart to stop working.

There may also be some additional benefits to the use of some diuretics which might support a claim of therapeutic use. The systemic diuretic acetazolamide appears to reduce mountain sickness and improve exercise performance at high altitude. Research suggests it can also produce an alkaline urine and so decrease the urinary output of some drugs for short periods of time; however, drugs remained in the urine for longer.

Probenecid has also been used by athletes in an attempt to mask the presence of drugs or their metabolites because of its ability to inhibit movement of molecules across kidney tissue. Use of probenecid first came to light in the Delgado affair, suspicions were alerted when a treatment for gout appeared in the urine of a seemingly healthy, active cyclist in competition. The combination of gas chromatography and mass spectrometry in the analytical procedure ensures that probenecid use no longer prevents detection.

## PEPTIDE HORMONES AND ANALOGUES

The increasing availability of hormone substances has led to greater use by athletes. Moreover the difficulties in detecting levels of abuse make them an attractive drug for athletes subject to testing. Corticotrophin (ACTH) increases adrenal corticosteroid levels in the body. The powerful antiinflammatory action of corticosteroids may be a useful aid to recovery from injury. Athletes might also seek the testicular stimulatory function of the gonadotrophins as a way to counter androgenic anabolic steroid effects.

Growth hormone would be used, presumably, for its

anabolic properties to increase size, strength or ultimate height, depending on the age of the user. As an injectable drug, there are risks associated with shared needles and syringes. Prior to the availability of synthetic growth hormone, use of cadaver pituitary gland infected with the Creutzfeldt-Jakob virus led to the development of Creutzfeldt-Jakob disease. Athletes are also using amino acid supplements in an attempt to stimulate their own growth hormone production, this is not currently prohibited.

Erythropoietin (EPO) is a peptide hormone which is used by athletes. Usually released from the kidney, EPO has more recently become more readily available due to recombinant DNA technology. EPO is the major hormone regulator of red blood cell production, used in medicine in cases of kidney failure. The long-term effects of use in medicine or misuse in sport are unknown, however overload of the cardiovascular system is likely where there is no medical need.

## BLOOD DOPING

Blood doping is a unique form of performance enhancement, as it does not involve the administration of drugs. Red blood cells or blood products containing red blood cells are administered intravenously in an attempt to gain unfair advantage in competition. The intravenous administration of red blood cells (either from the same individual or from a different but blood-type matched person) would increase the oxygen-carrying capacity of the blood. Competitors in endurance activities such as marathon and longdistance running, cycling and skiing might use blood doping to increase the oxygen-carrying capacity of the blood. Similar effects are reported from training at altitude.

Blood doping carries considerable risk to the athlete. Injection of an additional volume of blood can overload the cardiovascular system and induce metabolic shock. The use of an athlete's own blood can be safer in terms of cross-infection; however, adverse effects can be compounded if blood from a second individual is used. There may be a potentially fatal haemolytic reaction with kidney failure resulting from mismatched blood or allergic reaction. There is also an increased risk of contracting infectious diseases such as AIDS or viral hepatitis.

An alternative method of increasing blood haemoglobin and/or haematocrit is the use of erythropoietin (EPO).

## BETA BLOCKERS AND OTHER DRUGS WITH SEDATIVE ACTION

Among the range of drugs which may be misused are those whose actions are the opposite to the stimulant drugs. Certain sports require a steady action and an ability to control movements, such as archery and shooting.

If an athlete was seeking a drug which might help to improve performance, where a steady action was required, beta blockers have the potential to enhance this type of performance. By moderating the cardiac output and muscle blood flow caused by the nervous system's response to stress and arousal, beta blockers would generally reduce ability to perform strenuous physical sports. However, one of the side-effects noted in the treatment of cardiac arrhythmias was an ability to reduce muscle tremor. This would be of benefit in accuracy events and those where extraneous movement had to be kept under control.

The inclusion of beta blockers in the list of doping classes has not been without controversy. Their primary therapeutic use is in diseases of the cardiovascular system, due to their actions in reducing heart rate and cardiac output. This cardiodepressant effect can be useful. However, other side-effects such as cold hands and sleep disturbances may militate against their use in sport.

It is significant that early attempts to monitor their use were made by requiring a declaration of the medications and a doctor's certificate stating the reasons why they were required. At the 1984 Los Angeles Olympics, team doctors came forward with certificates to cover the whole team. The inclusion of beta blockers on the list of doping classes in 1985 was only one method to control their misuse. Officials in the sport of modern pentathlon tried to amend the competition timetable to hold the shooting event on the same day as the cross-country event. It was hoped that although beta blockers might be an advantage for the shooting event, they would be a positive disadvantage for running. In response, athletes simply moved to beta blockers with a shorter life which were metabolized before the running event began.

Fears that beta blockers may be misused in professional snooker have led to their inclusion on the list, but under pressure to address cases of medical need, the World Professional Billiards and Snooker Association have taken the unusual step of permitting, under certain circumstances and with prior permission, the use of cardioselective beta blockers for a heart condition. Applications for consent may require an independent medical examination and presentation of the full medical history. The introduction of this procedure reflects a growing trend towards acceptance of therapeutic drugs but a need to maintain control over potential misuse.

Beta blockers were moved to the 'Classes of drugs subject to certain restrictions' section of the IOC list in 1993, to indicate their specific application to certain sports. The IOC have also listed those Olympic sports where this restriction would be applicable (archery, shooting, biathlon, modern pentathlon, bobsleigh, diving, luge, ski-jumping). Debate as to whether beta blockers are prohibited for the sport of bowls has been inconclusive. Modern pentathlon has also tried to control the misuse of other sedative drugs such as barbiturates, benzodiazepines and antihistamines with sedative properties. The International Federation for Archery (FITA) have also introduced tighter controls on these drugs.

Obviously there are difficulties in trying to separate therapeutic use from misuse. With the increasing emphasis on scientific support for athletes, it is now possible to control anxiety without the use of drugs, calling on mental rehearsal and relaxation techniques.

## Local Anaesthetics

Local anaesthetics are permitted provided their use is medically justified, if the route of administration is either local or intra-articular. Cocaine is not permitted. In an attempt to control their misuse, details of the diagnosis, dose and route of administration must be submitted, in writing, to the IOC Medical Commission or Sports Federation. Local anaesthetics may be used to treat local injury but their use to block pain to enable an athlete to continue participating beyond the normal pain barrier is to be deprecated. There is a high risk of greater injury if the body's normal pain threshold is masked.

## CORTICOSTEROIDS

Corticosteroids are potent anti-inflammatory substances. In their naturally occurring form they are released by the adrenal gland during stress activity. The synthetically produced versions are used in medicine as analgesics and anti-inflammatories. In addition, corticosteroids are used in the treatment of asthma, a disease characterized by inflammation of the respiratory tract. Athletes seeking to open up the airways or, in larger doses, to mask injury or to increase training ability might misuse corticosteroids. They should not be confused with anabolic steroids.

Serious toxic effects can occur if corticosteroid use is prolonged or under inadequate medical control. Topical administration of corticosteroids is used in medicine wherever possible in preference to systemic treatment as adverse side-effects are less likely. Originally the IOC attempted to restrict their use in competition by requiring a declaration from doctors. However, because it became known that corticosteroids were being used non-therapeutically by the oral, rectal, intramuscular and even the intravenous route in some sports, stronger measures were introduced. The use of corticosteroids is now prohibited except for topical use (aural, ophthalmological and dermatological), inhalation therapy (asthma, allergic rhinitis) and local or intra-articular injections. Written notification must be given to the IOC Medical Commission or the sports federation.

### Alcohol

For most sports the use of alcohol would be detrimental

to performance, so it is logical that alcohol falls into the category of 'Classes of drugs subject to certain restrictions'. In low doses, alcohol (or ethanol) has some sedative effects. Higher doses can cause poor co-ordination, increased reaction time and mental confusion.

As a potential doping substance to reduce anxiety, the dose would have to be carefully controlled. In sports such as archery or shooting, the use of alcohol may stabilize tremor but could adversely affect reaction time and increase the unsteadiness of the arm when aiming. Because of the degree of euphoria alcohol can produce, it might also be used to overcome nervousness in other sports such as motor racing. Alcohol is also restricted for referees and umpires at international volleyball competitions.

## Pharmacological, Chemical or Physical Manipulation

As the testing programmes to control the use of doping substances have increased in sophistication, one response from athletes has been to try to manipulate the test in some way; the purpose being to invalidate the sample given or to secure the collection of a clean sample. Athletes have attempted to use other substances like vinegar to influence the quality of the urine. More often an athlete would try to provide a clean urine sample which had been obtained from another person during the procedure.

The clean sample is then secreted around the body and voided in place of the athlete's own urine. Tightening of the collection procedures, particularly in relation to the time between notification and collection of the sample have helped to control this practice. The collection procedures have also been challenged by an individual masquerading as the athlete presenting themselves for testing.

Checks on the identity and confirmation by official documentation are the only way to control this. Other forms of physical manipulation involve collusion between the athletes and the officials in the safe custody of the samples, the analysis of the samples at a laboratory which is not subject to independent monitoring or the manipulation of results.

Rumours of these forms of manipulation were noted in several governmental or sports federation inquiries into drug abuse in sport. Evidence of state-controlled drug-taking programmes, with and without the knowledge of the participants has emerged from former Eastern European countries.

It is sometimes difficult to justify scientifically why a substance has been included in the list of doping classes, it is not always for performance enhancement reasons. Many of the drugs which appear could possibly be removed; however, one of the complexities is that in the minds of athletes the drugs do work. A further complication is the tendency for athletes to engage in polypharmacy and supplementation emphasizing the belief that there are drugs which will improve performance, and that more is better.

## ATTITUDES TOWARDS DRUGS IN SPORT

The overwhelming majority of athletes I know would do anything, and take anything, short of killing themselves to improve athletic performance. There are many reasons why an athlete may take a drug, other than for legitimate therapeutic purposes. Previous experiences, at school or college, may prompt further experimentation with drugs within a sporting context. This approach may easily be fuelled by an athlete reading about drugs and their effects in popular magazines or even in serious scientific journals. Unfortunately, too many people involved in sport, at all levels, are prepared to speculate through television, newspapers or other media on the problem of drug abuse in sport.

Too often these unsubstantiated reports lead to accusations and counter-accusations between those involved in the practice and administration of sport. Such activities do little to enhance the reputation of sport and inevitably lead to confusion in the minds of the majority of sportsmen and women who do not take 'performance-enhancing' drugs. This uncertainty presents the greatest danger to those younger athletes who either become disenchanted with their chosen sport or are misled into believing that drug taking has become a necessary part of the route to sporting success.

Other athletes may experience pressure from peer groups, particularly fellow athletes from their own or other sports. This pressure may result from a desire to conform with the 'in-crowd'. Alternatively, it may be a fear of competing, on unequal terms, with athletes who are suspected of taking drugs. Peer pressure may also be exerted through fellow athletes encouraging an individual to participate in drug taking. Certainly drugs have become readily available and black market prices ensure that drug peddlers can make a handsome profit at the expense of athletes.

A different type of psychological pressure may be involved in another group of athletes. For these athletes, drug taking may be the last resort for the improvement of performance, having reached their apparent limit of capability by conventional methods of training.

The motivating factors for drug misuse do not necessarily lie in the hands of the athlete. It is an unfortunate fact that certain athletes are coerced into taking drugs by someone in authority. This person may be their coach, trainer or team doctor. The directive may even have originated from a country's governing body. Such pressures are obviously extremely difficult to resist, particularly where team selection is at stake. Evidence of the direct involvement of the government in the German Democratic Republic demonstrated not only the complicity of those in positions of trust but also the way the athletes themselves, in particular females, unknowingly took substances and have suffered the consequences.

Many studies have been carried out using questionnaires to ascertain attitudes towards drugs in sport. From these studies, the majority of athletes, coaches, medical practitioners and others involved in sport do not favour the use of performance-enhancing drugs. However, these results may reflect the respondent's ethical and moral attitudes to the problem, but in practice the pressures of competition may compel them to take a more pragmatic approach to drug taking. This denial of drug taking is a common feature among alcohol and drug abusers and further hinders any attempt at tackling the problem. Potentially more damaging is the type of athlete who openly admits to taking drugs and by so doing provides a model for the younger, more impressionable athletes to follow.

The blame for taking drugs does not, of course, always lie entirely with the athlete. There is often a body of so-called 'enablers' such as friends, family, and coaches who either actively encourage the athlete to participate in drug taking or vehemently shield the user from the need to deal with the problem. The reasons for this attitude are not always clear but in most cases involve self-interest. Conversely, those closely associated with the athlete may be unaware of their drug-abusing habits. This may, to a large extent, be due to a lack of knowledge and understanding of the drugs used and of their pharmacological effects.

It is clear that the majority of those involved in sport, both administrators and participants, are against the misuse of drugs in sport. It is equally clear that there is too little understanding of both the motivating factors that lead an athlete to take drugs and also the effects that those drugs can induce. It is vital that a wider knowledge of drugs and their adverse effects is achieved so that the current problem of drug abuse in sport can be contained and that future generations can be educated and persuaded against such misuse.

## Ethical Issues Associated with Drug Use in Sport

the use of doping agents in sport is both unhealthy and contrary to the ethics of sport, ...it is necessary to protect the physical and spiritual health of athletes, the values of fair play and of competition, the integrity and unity of sport, and the rights of those who take part in it at whatever level.

Drug use in sport is contrary to the very principles upon which sport is based. Sport is considered as character building, teaching 'the virtues of dedication, perseverance, endurance and self-discipline'. If, as Justice Dubin observes: 'sport helps us to learn from defeat as much as from victory, and team sports foster a spirit of co-operation and interdependence ...import(ing) something of moral and social values and...integrating us as individuals, to bring about a healthy, integrated society' drug abuse would have no place in sport. Justice Dubin goes on to ask 'how has it come about, then, that many athletes have resorted to cheating. Why are the rules that govern sport often regarded as obstacles to be overcome or circumvented rather than as regulations designed to create equality of competitive opportunity and to define the parameters of the sport?'

Using drugs in sport for the purpose of gaining an unfair advantage presents an ethical dilemma for athletes, coaches, doctors and officials. It is clearly cheating, moreover it may put the health of the athlete at risk. Furthermore it may also be calculated cheating, when quantities and substances are carefully monitored in an attempt to cheat the rules on drug testing. It has been argued that the ethical dilemma has emerged for many reasons:

- Media pressure to win;
- The prevalent attitude that doping is necessary to be successful;
- Public expectations about national competitiveness;
- Huge financial rewards of winning;
- The desire to be the best in the world;
- Performance-linked payments to athletes from Governments and sponsors;
- Coaching which emphasizes winning as the only goal;
- Unethical practices condoned by national and international sports federations;
- Competitive character of the athlete;
- Infallibility of the 'medical' profession to cure and improve performance;
- Psychological belief in aids to performance-the magic pill;
- The development of spectator sport; and
- A crowded competition calendar.

The majority of these reasons were cited in the Dubin Inquiry itself, as explanations were sought for the context in which five Canadian athletes (four weightlifters and one track and field athlete) came to be disqualified for anabolic steroid use at the Seoul Olympics. René Maheu has noted that development of spectator sport has turned attention away from the moral value of sport for the individual towards its entertainment potential. 'The success of spectator sport and the importance it has come to assume in everyday life are unfortunately too often exploited for purposes alien to or even opposed to sport-commercialism, chauvinism and politics-which corrupt and deform it.'

Dubin, however, whilst acknowledging the existence of all the influences and their undoubted effects which might lead to drug misuse in sport, argued first that there can be no justification for athletes to cheat in order to win, and second that the pressures and temptations are the same for all athletes yet most show greater character and do not succumb. He concluded the problem is not educational, economic or social but, essentially, a moral problem.

The sporting contest is seen to have been replaced by a competition between doctors and biochemists on the one side and the regulating authorities on the other. The athlete becomes the puppet of this technology, health risks are simply ignored and other competitors cannot participate in the competition unless they, too, are prepared to use substances to improve performance. In an era where genetic and chemical manipulation has become commonplace it is hardly surprising that some athletes no longer rely on their natural abilities and skills.

In 1892 at a conference at the Sorbonne, Baron de Coubertin, founder of the modern Olympics said: 'Before all things it is necessary that we should preserve in sport these characteristics of nobility and chivalry which have distinguished it in the past, so that it may continue to play the same part in the education of the peoples of today as it played so admirably in the days of ancient Greece.'

This may have been so at the turn of the twentieth century and the emergence of the modern day Olympic Games, yet in present day sport, the pressures on all concerned are immense. An athlete is faced with the pressures of winning, of competing, of meeting the expectations of the coach, team-mates, family and friends. Coaches are under pressure to produce the winning combination, of coping with fitness levels and of making demands on individual competitors, which may give the wrong signals in respect of drug misuse. Doctors may be faced with the dilemma of prescribing drugs for athletes and monitoring their effects as a safe way of containing drug misuse rather than know an athlete will seek black market sources and advice. The doping regulations may also apply to others who assist or incite an athlete to commit a doping offence.

Occasionally, criticisms of the drug-testing procedure itself are made: in particular the suggestion of invasion of privacy and impropriety in observing a person urinating. Athletes are looking forward to the advent of blood testing as a sophisticated progression towards comprehensive doping control. However, it is likely to be some time before scientists are willing to move from urine analysis because of the range of substances which can be detected. Blood testing offers a limited opportunity for detection of prohibited substances at present.

There is also another perspective, that of 'what constitutes drug misuse?'. Some banned substances actually originate in the body and it is an excessive level which has been deemed to be a doping offence. Critics would argue this level has been arbitrarily set. Other substances, such as ephedrine and caffeine, commonly occur in over-the-counter medications, herbal preparations and even in social drinks. Do they actually improve performance? There is no doubt that athletes are prepared to make use of these substances to assist their performance. In terms of drugs with a therapeutic purpose there is also considerable abuse of medications by athletes who have no therapeutic indication. Given this array of drug misuse by sportsmen and women, it is hardly surprising that anti-doping rules have been introduced.

The definition of doping has to begin somewhere. The time may have come for the critics and the sports regulators to work together to achieve a practical set of rules, a realistic competitive calendar, an efficient support system and greater controls on the commercialization of sport. Elite athletes have become the focus of a considerable amount of media attention, with stories about their injuries and illnesses filling column inches.

Moreover, speculation and reporting about the lifestyle of professional athletes has given rise to an image totally out of step with the dedication, training and motivation required to survive the sporting calendar. In many sports, increasing commercialism has seen a price put on an athlete's head; some cope better with this than others.

## AN INTERNATIONAL POLICY PERSPECTIVE/ GOVERNMENT ACTION AND POLICY

Drug use and abuse by athletes has now become a frequent feature of sport. It is clear that if drug use and abuse in sport is to be treated seriously it will require consolidated action, a joint commitment by sport, governments and others. In the words of Justice Dubin 'The resolution of this problem cannot simply be left to those who govern sport nationally and internationally.'

Initially, sport attempted to put its own house in order, and it was the international sports federations and the IOC who were the first bodies to introduce testing. Concern that the commitment required to achieve effective controls was lacking led to the involvement of governments. Testing had been limited to major competitions such as the Olympic Games and world championships; the regulations of the international sports federations introduced testing in a limited way. The IOC created a reference list of prohibited substances and proceeded to amend it to reflect doping practices. Testing programmes rested on accurate analysis.

The IAAF and the IOC undertook the accreditation of laboratories for the analysis of urine samples. In many ways the progress being made to control drug misuse was not sufficient to demonstrate a real commitment to resolving the problem. The limitations and potential conflicts of interest which developed in the way testing programmes were delivered did nothing to reassure governments that action taken was sufficient and others began to take a close interest in the control of drugs in sport.

Governments became the other key players in the fight against doping. Sport is played on a national level throughout the world and governments were concerned about the ineffectiveness of the inconsistent actions of sports bodies, some had regulations-some did not. In 1967, prior to the first testing at an Olympic Games, the Committee of Ministers of the Council of Europe adopted a resolution on doping in sport, the first international text of its kind. The resolution stressed the moral and ethical principles at stake for sport, and the health dangers for athletes.

The resolution explicitly referred to doping as cheating and included a broad definition of doping, including doping methods as well as the misuse of drugs. Governments were recommended to persuade sports organizations to take the necessary steps to have proper and adequate regulations and to penalize offenders. Finally the resolution recommended governments to take action themselves if the sports organization did not act sufficiently within 3 years. Anti-doping legislation was introduced in several European countries in response to this resolution.

Having continued to monitor the situation for 11 years, sports ministers adopted a further resolution in 1978, which called for governments to provide a co-ordinated policy and an overall framework in which the doping controls of sports organizations could take place. A European Charter, a statement of principles, anti-doping strategies and policies was adopted in 1984.

It is significant that the chairman of the drafting group was the Chairman of the IOC Medical Commission, Prince Alexandre de Merode and that the Charter received the support from international sports organizations. It was obvious that sport alone would be unable to contain the problem; the Charter provided the first opportunity for governments to drive the agenda with the sports bodies, many of whom appeared to be above the law in the way they dealt with doping matters.

Although the Charter received support from international sports organizations it was not binding upon governments, but would have 'moral, political and practical impact'.

Anxious to keep up the momentum, the Council of Europe Committee of Ministers pressed for testing out of competition without prior warning to the athlete. Ministers also sought to secure a commitment to international harmonization, not only among sports but also among countries. Ministers agreed to the drafting of an anti-doping convention in 1989 that would be binding on governments.

The key significance of this document was the recognition of political will to address the problem of doping. The Convention also provides a number of common standards-legislative, financial, technical and education, for implementation by all the bodies concerned with the state, by governments themselves and by government in support of sports organizations. Governments have embraced the standards being agreed through the Convention, although not wholeheartedly supported by the international sports organizations. In some countries the Convention has been adopted as the national legislation.

Progress towards a uniform international anti-doping policy took a further step forward when the IOC, international sports organizations and national governments came together at the First Permanent World Conference on Anti-Doping in 1988. The outcome of this conference was the development of the International Olympic Charter against Doping in Sport. This important document identified the policies and practices required to counter doping and was relevant mainly to national policies and practice. Its adoption as an IOC Charter was crucial to its success and influence, although the full support of the sports movement was not evidenced in the anti-doping programmes of that time.

A second world conference the following year in Moscow helped to take forward some practical issues such as the operating standards for out-of-competition testing. However, a third world conference in London in 1993 focusing on the planning of testing programmes, national organization of anti-doping programmes, ethics and education showed the broader agenda still in need of attention. After that conference the sport/government partnership appeared to falter.

Whilst recognition of the need for a symbiotic relationship between sports organizations and governments was noted in the IOC/IF Agreement against Doping in Sport in June 1993, the identification of roles may be illustrative of underlying tensions. In seeking ways to 'intensify the prevention of, education and fight against doping in sport', the IOC and International Sports Federations agreed to 'develop the co-operation between the IOC, The International Sports Federations, the National Olympic Committees, the National Federations and the governmental or other organizations concerned in order to combat the trafficking of doping substances'.

Interestingly, International Sports Federations were invited 'to adopt each year as a basic minimum document, the list of banned classes and methods established by the IOC Medical Commission and to undertake the appropriate controls for each sport'. Sport was clearly indicating the role for governments in the regulation of supply and availability of drugs, whilst reserving the actual controls in sport for the sports movement.

In the 1990s actions to control drug misuse in sport were numerous. Initially the IOC took control of the doping in sport agenda. Harmonization was the theme of a conference called in Lausanne in 1994 for the IOC Associations of Summer and Winter Olympic Federations, National Olympic Committees and athlete representatives and led to the publication of more unified rules and procedures in the document Preventing and fighting against doping in sport.

The very next year the IOC published the IOC Medical Code, bringing together the IOC anti-doping rules and regulations in one document for the first time in 1995. However, the sports federations were slow to adopt the IOC standards, and differences in the lists of prohibited substances, the sanctions to be applied, and waiver in respect of minor procedural irregularities were evident. The compilation of directories of international sports federations' anti-doping regulations by UK Sport demonstrated that essential differences between sports remained, notably in the definition of doping itself.

Governments have continued to be critical of the lack of action by sports organizations themselves to address the problem seriously from within. In 1987 the then UK Sports Minister Colin Moynihan and former Olympic athlete Sebastian Coe co-authored a report that noted 'Within the present arrangements there appear to be too many loopholes, and perhaps insufficient security for satisfactory levels of effectiveness and confidence to be achieved ...there is too much potential for evasion, leading to public concern and also to frustration among administrators and sportsmen and women.'

Similarly the Commission of Inquiry into the Use of Drugs and Banned Practices intended to Increase Athletic Performance in Canada in 1990 pointed to the failure of leadership among sports organizations and to the involvement and compliance of officials in drug use. The evidence of those witnesses at this inquiry who admitted their use of banned substances was in large part instrumental in uncovering the scandalous and pervasive practice of doping in sport that until then has hidden from public view, although not from the view of national and international sports federations.'

The action taken by sport itself, whilst an important contribution, can only be strengthened by a concerted world-wide effort supported by governments. Regrettably there have also been incidents of testing programmes actually being used to cover-up drug misuse.

Testing of athletes prior to a major event to determine whether they would pass the competition test has been admitted in several former Eastern bloc countries. Covering-up results from major competitions has also been revealed. Robert Voy, formerly Chief Medical Officer to the United States Olympic Committee explained how problematic this is: 'Allowing National Governing Bodies (NGBs), International Federations

(IFs) and National Olympic Committees (NOCs) such as the United States Olympic Committee to govern the testing process to ensure fair play in sport is terribly ineffective. In a sense it is like having the fox guard the hen house'. Independence of the testing programmes and an openness of information would seem to be the only way forward, if public confidence and in particular the confidence of athletes is to be restored.

It is significant that the IOC's own role at that time indirectly extended outside the Olympic Games through the accreditation of laboratories, the establishment of the list of doping classes, a financial assistance programme for IFs who need help to intensify their anti-doping controls and encouragement to Olympic sports to comply with the principles of the agreement. Yet their role was dogged with suggestions and innuendos about conflicts of interest, even direct actions to cover-up doping issues within the Olympic family.

Co-operation between international and national sports federations and the newly created national anti-doping organizations has the potential to provide one of the strongest practical deterrents to drug misuse. However, the authority of international sports federations and of national policies and legislation can sometimes lie uneasily together. Some sports have interpreted the intervention of governments in anti-doping matters as threatening their independence and challenging their abilities to undertake urine sampling. As the majority of testing and especially laboratory expertise is government funded, a mutually supportive relationship between sports organizations and governments is crucial to the ongoing success of anti-doping activities.

The response of governments and international organizations to the whole issue of doping in sport has been significant and interesting. Government-initiated enquiries in Australia, Canada, New Zealand and the UK have acted as a catalyst for progress in anti-doping activities, creating the International Anti-Doping Arrangement (IADA), in 1990, an intergovernmental agreement on consolidated actions in the fight against drug misuse. Originally founded by the countries of Australia, Canada and the UK, this alliance was soon joined by the countries of Norway, New Zealand, Sweden, Netherlands, Denmark and Finland.

At about the same time the Nordic Convention between the Scandinavian countries opened up the borders to reciprocal testing and mutual recognition of results, working directly with their sports federations, sometimes adopting a stronger position than the international federation. The strong alliance of the IADA countries has led to the achievement of the most significant development in standardization of anti-doping procedures, the International Standard for Doping Control, a quality assured standard for the planning, implementation and monitoring of results of testing. Several international forums have now endorsed this standard as the accepted standard for anti-doping programmes and the International Standards Organization are presently considering its transfer to an ISO certified standard.

In an article published in 1992, the Chairman of the IOC Medical Commission acknowledged the strategy of a common policy to be the most effective, he stated: 'A commonly accepted international policy is necessary for the elimination of doping in sport. Such a policy would lead to an improved and more consistent approach and would contribute to equality and equity in the international sporting community. Both public authorities and the independent sports organizations have separate but complimentary responsibilities and should work together for this purpose at all levels.'

Legislation has become a major problem for sport as athletes turned to the law to address perceived inconsistencies in the rules of sport, Katrin Krabbe, Harry Reynolds and Diane Modahl were only some of the high profile cases that challenged the reliability of testing procedures and resulted in significant financial pressure upon the national federations. Governments also added to the pressures by making funding of sport conditional upon minimum anti-doping programmes, as required by the 1989 Anti-Doping Convention, which was gathering speed as more countries adopted its articles into their national policies and laws. In some countries the requirements for an effective anti-doping response were enforced through legislation. The direct action taken by the French Government to intervene during the 1998 Tour de France and reveal evidence of blood doping and drug misuse shocked the sporting world but won the admiration of athletes.

The International Cycling Federation, previously considered one of the more responsible federations in anti-doping procedures, was exposed as failing to address the extensive drug misuse in this premier event. These events were undoubtedly the catalyst for the IOC response in February the following year.

The ongoing tensions surrounding the allegations of cover-ups in the testing at the 1996 Atlanta Games, the scandals of corruption and bribery over Olympic bidding and increasing interest of the European Union to intervene more directly culminated in the most significant opportunity for drug-free sport finally to become a possibility. In 1999 the IOC called a World Conference on Anti-Doping in Sport in Lausanne. This conference attended by sports federations and the IOC also attracted a number of government ministers. In particular the Director of the United States Office on National Drug Control Policy Barry McCaffrey and UK Sports Minister Tony Banks were vociferous in their criticism of the IOC. Support for a new independent world agency spread and was evident among many of the athletes and sports federations present.

The debate demonstrated the strength of feeling among the governments to require the sports movement to clean up their sports or face government intervention. Initial suggestions to form an international anti-doping agency, 'headquartered in Lausanne, governed by a council presided over by the IOC President' were rejected. The conference culminated in an agreement to form the World Anti-Doping Agency, 'to be fully operational in time for the XXVII Olympiad in Sydney in 2000' as an equal partnership between sport and governments.

In the years following there has been an uneasy struggle to find a basis for the formal establishment and operation of the World Anti-Doping Agency (WADA) in a way that would ensure mutual ownership but not surrender control to either sport or government. The IOC originally offered funding with an expectation that governments would pay their share and the bidding process for a permanent home began in earnest. The government side has developed regional co-ordination across the world under the umbrella of the 'International Intergovernmental Consultative Group on Anti-Doping'. Meetings have been held in Montreal, Oslo, Cape Town and Kuala Lumpur involving an increasing number of governments in the fight against doping.

WADA has sought greater legitimacy in promoting drug-free sport. Among its responsibilities are 'expanding out of competition testing, co-ordinating research, promoting preventive and educational actions and harmonizing scientific and technical standards and procedures for analyses and equipment'. WADA programme of testing out of competition has been initiated through a contracted arrangement with a consortium of government-sponsored national anti-doping agencies. Debate about the additional testing in countries where there are strong independent national programmes has led to some criticism of WADA's ability to meet its principal objectives. Duplication of testing by international federations and national agencies as well as the Australian government prior to the Sydney Olympics demonstrated the need for greater co-ordination, although the question of who would give up the authority to test remains a vexed question. The Sydney Olympics marked a turning point in the accountability for testing under the control of the IOC, when the WADA observer programme was introduced.

Unexpectedly, the voting of the Foundation Board led to the WADA headquarters being located in Montreal. The offices opened in April 2002. Further work is continuing on the development of a WADA Framework and Code. If agreed, this should provide the basis for a symbiotic relationship between sport and government. Early indications are that compliance could be linked to eligibility to participate in Olympic Games and to host world championships.

## Chapter 3

# Central Nervous System Stimulants

Various drugs which stimulate the central nervous system (CNS) have been known for over 2000 years. A simple classification of these substances is complicated by their combination of central and systemic effects. Thus, though the compounds mainly stimulate CNS activity, many central stimulants have, in addition, direct effects on cardiovascular functions and on the sympathetic nervous system.

## CNS NEUROPHYSIOLOGY

To understand the various mechanisms by which CNS stimulants produce their effects, it is necessary to understand the basic functioning of neurones in the CNS. The stimulant drug must pass from the circulation, across the blood-brain barrier and into the brain tissue spaces. Once in the brain it may: (a) increase neurotransmitter release on to receptors (e.g. amphetamine and ephedrine); (b) directly stimulate the post-synaptic receptors (e.g. ephedrine and caffeine); or (c) inhibit neurotransmitter re-uptake (e.g. cocaine and amphetamine).

CNS stimulants are thought to act mainly on the dopamine (DA), noradrenaline (NA) and 5-hydroxytryptamine (5HT) (serotonin) neurotransmitter systems. Caffeine is thought to affect adenosine neurotransmission.

## AMPHETAMINES

Several structurally related drugs are known as 'amphetamines' and include dextroamphetamine, methamphetamine, phenmetrazine and methylphenidate. Amphetamine is a phenyl isopropylamine and was first synthesized in 1920. It was originally prescribed for the treatment of nasal congestion-inhalation of an amphetamine spray through the nose induced

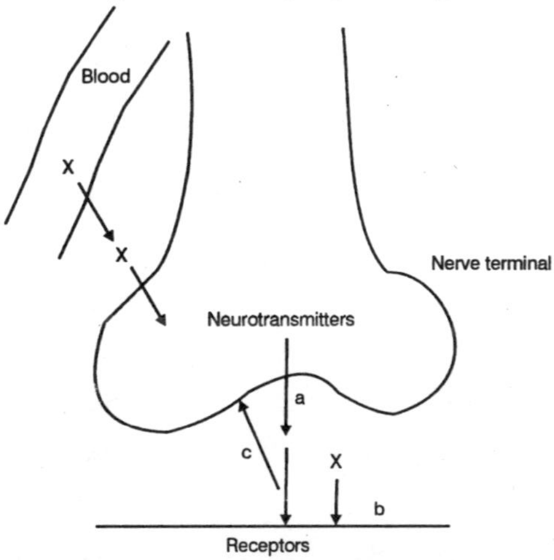


**Fig.** Sites of Action of CNS Stimulants (a) Amphetamines; (b) Caffeine; (c) Amphetamine and Cocaine.

nasal vasoconstriction which resulted in decongestion. Amphetamine was first used to treat the neurological condition narcolepsy, and its use in the treatment of depression, anxiety and hyperactivity in children followed from this. Amphetamine was used widely during the Second World War to reduce fatigue and increase alertness, particularly amongst naval and airforce crew on patrol duties. Reference to this was made in 1974 in Ludovic Kennedy's account of the pursuit and sinking of the German battleship Bismarck. The rapid development of tolerance to amphetamine and the insidious occurrence of dependence have led to the drug being withdrawn from clinical use, except in certain controlled circumstances, in both Britain and the USA.

## The effect of Amphetamines on Human Mood and Performance

The desire to enhance mood or performance or both is usually the main reason for taking amphetamines. In their comprehensive review of amphetamines Weiss and Laties agreed that amphetamine does produce an enhanced performance in many tasks and does not simply normalize fatigue responses.

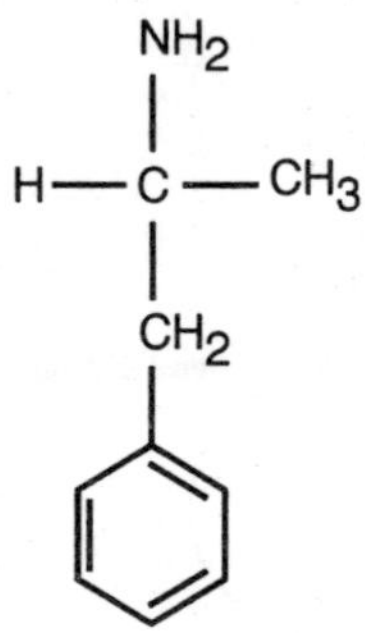

Amphetamines

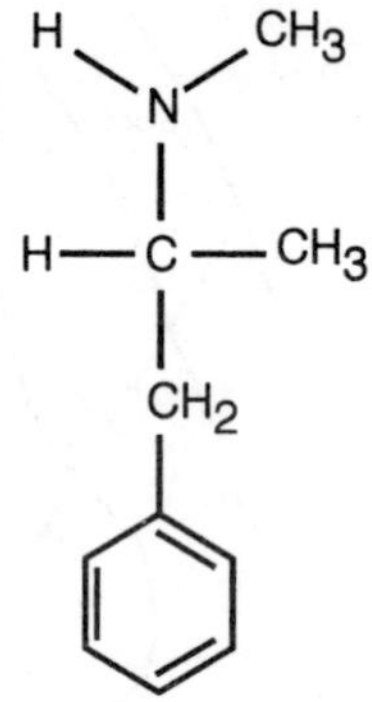

Methamphetamines

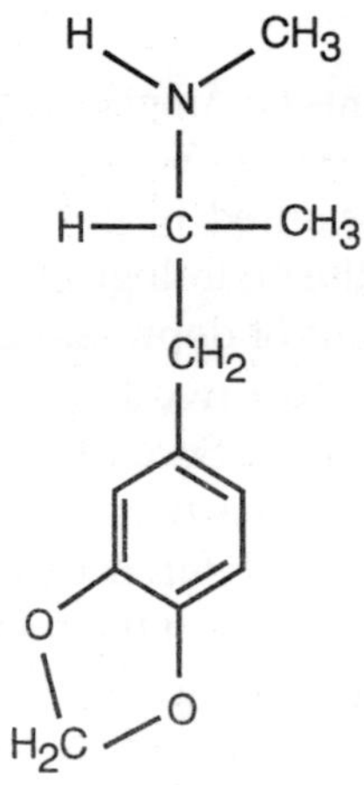

Ecstaag

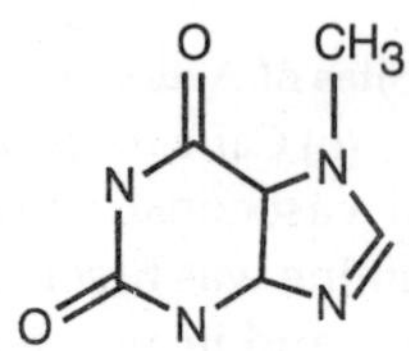

Caffeine

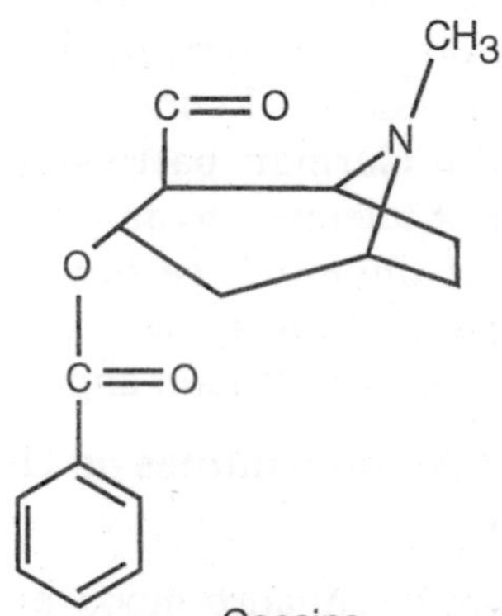

Cocaine

**Fig.** Some Central Stimulants.

They examined various tasks such as (a) work output by subjects on a bicycle ergometer, (b) Performance on arduous military exercises, and (c) Performance during flying or driving missions. Apparent improvements in athletic performance in events as diverse as shot put, swimming and running are produced by amphetamines as well as a reduction in reaction time and increased co-ordination and steadiness. Intellectual performance does not seem to be improved by amphetamines, unless the performance has been degraded by boredom and fatigue. In the short term, amphetamine increases the speed of learning of new tasks.

The effects of amphetamine on judgement are uncertain and several conflicting studies have been published. There is general agreement that amphetamines cause a mild distortion of time perception which may lead to misjudgement in planning manoeuvres or in manipulations such as driving a car. Active avoidance learning is facilitated by amphetamine. Although there is considerable interindividual variation in the effects of amphetamine on mood, the general effects are of positive mood enhancement.

These positive effects include an increase in physical energy, mental aptitude, talkativeness, restlessness, vigour, excitement and good humour. Subjects taking amphetamine also report that they feel confident, efficient, ambitious and that their food intake is reduced. Many athletes report that they feel most aggressive when taking amphetamines and are unlikely to report or complain of injuries.

Some 'negative' effects of amphetamine include anxiety, indifference, slowness in reasoning, irresponsible behaviour, irritability and restlessness, dry mouth, tremors, insomnia and following withdrawal, depression. These effects of amphetamine on mood are dose-dependent and are thought to be produced by the stimulation of dopamine and adrenergic receptors.

## Tolerance and Dependence

Tolerance develops rapidly to many of the effects of the amphetamines. Tolerance is said to be present when, over a period of time, increasing doses of a drug are required to maintain the same response. Brookes has reported several cases of subjects requiring as much as 1 g of amphetamine per day to produce the same effect on mood as a new taker of amphetamines who may require only 10-30 mg.

There is much evidence to show that amphetamines induce drug dependence and the amphetamine-dependent person may become psychotic aggressive and anti-social. Withdrawal of amphetamines is associated with mental and physical depression. Recent evidence by Comer's group in New York suggests that tolerance to the positive effects of methamphetamine does occur over time at least in new abusers while the severity of the negative effects increases over time. Another study by the same group showed that methamphetamine is a powerful, positive reinforcing agent in humans as well as animals.

### Therapeutic use

The many varied uses of amphetamine following its original introduction are now largely discredited. It is interesting to compare the initial enthusiasm for amphetamine as the 'cure-all' for numerous mental problems with that for the use of cocaine some 50 years previously.

Until quite recently amphetamine was used to treat narcolepsy, but its use is now limited to the treatment of hyperactivity in children. A rare use of amphetamines is as a diagnostic aid in determining which patients are unsuitable for a particular anti-manic or anti-schizophrenic treatment.

## TOXICITY

The major side-effects of amphetamine administration (excluding those following withdrawal of the drug) include:

- Many of the negative effects described previously;
- Confusion, delirium, sweating, palpitations, dilation of the pupil and rapid breathing; and
- Hypertension, tachycardia, tremors, muscle and joint pain. Though amphetamines may initially stimulate libido, chronic amphetamine use often leads to a

reduction in sex drive. Chronic amphetamine administration is also associated with myocardial pathology and with growth retardation in adolescents. Usually the personality changes induced by chronic low doses of amphetamine are gradually reversed after the drug is stopped. However, high chronic doses may lead to a variety of persistent personality changes. Possibly the most serious of the severe psychiatric disorders induced by amphetamine is the so-called amphetamine psychosis described by Connell in 1958. The frightening array of psychiatric symptoms he described in patients presenting with amphetamine psychosis include many commonly found in paranoid-type schizophrenics. An important distinction between amphetamine psychosis and schizophrenia is that amphetamine induces a preponderance of symptoms of paranoid and of tactile hallucinations.

## THE MODE OF ACTION OF AMPHETAMINE

There are four mechanisms by which amphetamine may produce its effects. These are:

- Release of neurotransmitter-dopamine (DA), noradrenaline or 5HT-from their respective nerve terminals;
- Inhibition of monoamine oxidase activity;
- Inhibition of neurotransmitter re-uptake; and
- Direct action on neurotransmitter receptors. Of these four possibilities, neurotransmitter release appears to be the most important.

Amphetamine stimulates DA release by reversing the neuronal membrane uptake transporter. It also inhibits the activity of the enzyme monoamine oxidase. It seems that several major behavioural changes induced by amphetamine are most closely mimicked by stimulation of central noradrenaline-releasing neurones. Thus, the amphetamine-induced locomotor activity and self-stimulation seen in animals and the increased alertness and elevation of mood produced in humans are closely related to increases in noradrenergic activity. Amphetamine is a potent anorectic and elevates plasma free fatty acid levels. Body temperature is also elevated. The cardiovascular, gastrointestinal and respiratory effects of amphetamine are sympathomimetic in nature.

However, both animal and clinical experiments suggest that the effects of amphetamine are mediated by the release of at least two neurotransmitters, NA and DA, and that in the rat the development of tolerance to amphetamine involves the release of 5HT. However, the stereotyped behaviour induced in the rat by amphetamine administration appears to depend on DA release. The euphoriant action of amphetamine can be abolished by the DA receptor antagonists such as haloperidol and pimozide. There is some evidence to suggest that the positive behavioural effects of amphetamine may be mediated by DA while the effect of amphetamine on food intake may be mediated by NA. However, Silverstone and Goodall produced conflicting evidence of this.

### Pharmocokinetics

Amphetamines are readily absorbed, mainly from the small intestine and the peak plasma concentration occurs in 1-2 hours following administration. Absorption is usually complete in 2.5-4 hours and is accelerated by food intake.

The metabolism of amphetamines has been difficult to investigate because of the wide variation between species in the metabolic effects of amphetamines. The principal amphetamine metabolites are p-hydroxyephedrine and p-hydroxyamphetamine. Both these metabolites have similar pharmacological effects to the parent amphetamine. Amphetamine is lost from the blood by renal filtration. An acid urine and treatments which increase the acidity of urine enhance amphetamine loss-a reaction which is useful in the treatment of amphetamine overdose.

## THE EFFECTS OF AMPHETAMINES IN SPORT

In the USA, the increasing use of amphetamines in all sports led the American Medical Association to initiate research projects to test the effects of amphetamine on sports performance and the incidence of side-effects associated with the drug. One of these studies reported that 14-21 mg of amphetamine sulphate per kg body weight when administered 2-3 hours prior to running, swimming or weight throwing, improved performance in 75 per cent of the cases investigated.

This was a double-blind study in which 14 out of 15 swimmers and 19 out of 26 runners showed a statistically significant improvement in performance after amphetamine administration. However, the improvements demonstrated were quite small (usually 1 per cent).

This study also demonstrated that the performance of athletes in throwing events was improved by an average of 4 per cent following amphetamine administration. Criticism of the study soon followed because the athletes were sometimes allowed to time themselves, there was little control for weather conditions, a wide range of distances (600 yards to 12 miles) was used to test the athletes and a minor dosage of amphetamine was administered. Chandler and Blair reported that amphetamine improved athletic performance in terms of acceleration, knee extension strength and time to exhaustion but that it had no effect on sprinting speed.

Haldi and Wynn reported that 5 mg of amphetamine 90 minutes before a 100-yard swim had no effect on the time of the swim. A more sophisticated double-blind investigation of amphetamine was carried out by Golding and Barnard using a treadmill. They studied the effect of amphetamine on treadmill running in trained and untrained subjects. Each subject undertook an initial run followed 12 minutes later by a second 'fatigued' run. Thus, the effects of amphetamine on initial performance and fatigue could be examined in the same subject. Their subjects showed that amphetamine had no effect on performance during the initial and fatigued runs in either the trained or the untrained athletes.

During the fatigued runs, amphetamine retarded the recovery rates for heart rate and blood pressure. Only one of the subjects was able to tell that he was receiving amphetamine. Many of the studies on the effects of amphetamine on athletic performance have been carried out on cyclists. One reason for this is that there are numerous examples of fatalities arising from the use of amphetamines by cyclists, notably the incidence of death from heat-stroke. Wide-ranging placebo-controlled biochemical and physiological investigation on two champion cyclists exercising on a bicycle ergometer.

Whilst working at rates between 12000 and 16000 ft/lb.min there was no difference between amphetamine and placebo in terms of submaximal or maximal oxygen uptake, heart rate or minute ventilation; however, there were significant increases in blood lactate levels. The authors concluded that amphetamines have no effect on the ability to do aerobic work but they insignificantly increased the cyclists' ability to tolerate higher levels of anaerobic metabolism.

The dangers inherent in these results are that an athlete taking amphetamine might be better able to ignore the usual internal signals of over-exertion and heat stress, which may therefore explain the incidence of heat-stroke and cardiac problems in cyclists who take amphetamines during long-distance cycling events. This has been attributed to a decline in the abuse of amphetamine by athletes and by the general public, following increased controls on its prescription and availability.

Several reviewers, including Conlee have remarked on the considerable inconsistency of amphetamine effects in humans, particularly with regard to ergogenicity. A poorly explored feature of amphetamine action is its effect on fatigue. Most studies have concentrated on the central aspects of fatigue while neglecting peripheral contributions. However, the few studies of amphetamine effects on muscle glycogen stores before and during exercise have been contradictory.

Since no significant improvement in performance is associated with amphetamine use, why does it continue to be taken? The answer could be an effect on mental attitude in terms of improved mood, greater confidence and optimism and increased alertness. It should also be remembered that, like anabolic steroids amphetamine could be abused for different reasons by different athletes. Thus, baseball and football players may use them to increase alertness and concentration, runners or swimmers to increase energy and endurance.

An interesting insight into the differential abuse of amphetamine in an American football team has been provided by Mandell. They reported that amphetamine dosage would be adjusted according to the players' position in the team. The lowest doses of 5-15 mg per man per game were given to those players, such as wide receivers, whose concentration needed to be heightened while maintaining near normal perception. The high doses of 10-60 mg per man per game (line-backers) and 30-150 mg per man per game (defensive linemen) went to those players in whom aggression was paramount.

It is also possible that amphetamine might increase preparedness and make the athlete more keyed up for his event. To examine this possibility the effects of amphetamine sulphate were compared with the tranquillizer meprobamate and with placebo control in 126 male medical students. The results showed that none of the students was able to tell which drug he was taking and also there was no correlation between either subjective feelings of increased alertness in those taking amphetamine or lethargy in subjects on meprobamate, with any change in reaction time or manipulative skills.

Several studies thus indicate that the effect of amphetamine on the psychological state of athletes might be self-induced and occurs as a result of the athlete expecting to perform better and be more alert. These and other aspects plus confounding influences in psychostimulant results have been reviewed by Clarkson and Thompson. They quoted two studies carried out in the 1940s in which all the subjects on active drug (amphetamine) perceived that they had done more work on a cycle ergometer than was actually measured. In their review they also question the validity of some of the earlier experiments in terms of clinical methodological vigour (blindness), statistical inference and control. Several studies quoted have low numbers of participants and the detection of active drug by the subject was not controlled.

Another feature of most studies is the failure to control for trained or untrained subjects, a confounding feature of many anabolic steroid studies. This is very important if we are considering that amphetamine may have an effect on motivation, as trained athletes often exhibit higher motivational levels than the untrained and the untrained therefore may not exercise fully to exhaustion.

## SIDE-EFFECTS OF AMPHETAMINE IN RELATION TO SPORT

Some side-effects of amphetamine are particularly important in athletes and have often only been revealed in individuals undertaking extremely arduous training or sporting schedules. One of the most widely publicised side-effects of amphetamine from which a number of fatalities have occurred is heat-stroke. This has been most prominent in cyclists owing to the intensity of their exercise, the endurance required and the high ambient temperatures at which the exercise often occurs.

Amphetamine causes a redistribution of blood flow away from the skin, thus limiting the cooling of the blood. As a result of this, two cyclists who had both been taking amphetamine died of heat-stroke and cardiac arrest, respectively, during gruelling road races. The former occurred in the intense summer heat of Rome, the latter whilst climbing the infamous Mont Ventoux during the 1967 Tour de France.

The ability of amphetamines to obscure painful injuries has enabled many American footballers to play on and exacerbate injuries which would normally have resulted in their withdrawal from play, and soldiers to continue marching while they have foot blisters.

The side-effects of amphetamine on behaviour are also important in sport. Mandell has investigated amphetamine abuse amongst American footballers and found extensive abuse amounting to 60-70 mg average dose per man per game. In this sport, amphetamine was administered apparently to promote aggression and weaken fatigue in the footballers. However, there are several accounts quoted by Golding in which the euphoriant effects of such doses have rendered the takers unaware of the errors and misjudgements they were making on the pitch.

## Amphetamines

Why take amphetamines when the chance of increased injury, dependence, heat-stroke and cardiac arrest is enhanced by these drugs and the actual improvement on performance, if it does occur, is so small-in the order of 1 or 2 per cent? The simple answer to this was proposed by Laties and Weiss who examined the improvements in world records in athletic events over the past 100 years. As an example, the 1500 m world record has improved by only 15 per cent since 1880 and on average in the past 50 years it has improved by only 1 per cent in every 7 years.

Thus, they concluded that a top athlete who could consistently maintain a 1 per cent improvement in performance would be at an advantage over competitors. This advantage they termed 'the amphetamine margin'. The prescription and administration of amphetamines are strictly controlled by law in most developed countries. They produce powerful stimulating effects on the CNS, which include euphoria, excitation and increased aggression and alertness. These effects are achieved at the expense of judgement and self-criticism. Amphetamine administration may be followed by severe bouts of depression and dependence.

Increases in athletic performance induced by amphetamine are very small and several studies have failed to show that amphetamine produces any physical advantage. Some evidence suggests that amphetamine may increase confidence before and during an event, and laboratory studies have shown that it may also reduce fatigue in isometric muscle construction.

The induction of dependence and the increased susceptibility to heat-stroke and cardiac abnormalities seem to suggest that amphetamine taking is of little value as a performance-enhancing drug in the long term. The fact that amphetamine derivatives of lower potency, such as 1-

amphetamine, are still present in some OTC medications available overseas, should serve as a reminder to all those competition athletes seeking medication abroad. A recent mistake cost the UK skier Alain Baxter his Olympic bronze medal in 2002.

### Ecstasy

This is an amphetamine derivative and was synthesized as early as 1914, being used initially as an appetite suppressant. It has been a class A illegal substance since 1977 in the UK and a controlled drug in the USA since 1985. Ecstasy has amphetamine-like stimulant properties and is associated with increased stamina and endurance. Its abuse is most commonly associated with social activities such as dancing. However, it is described here because of its possible misuse by athletes, though since 1990, no cases of positive ecstasy tests have been reported in the UK.

Ecstasy produces its effects by stimulating the release of the neurotransmitter 5HT from 5HT-releasing neurones in the CNS and can induce the destruction of these neurones. Its most serious physical side-effects are hyperpyrexia, which is the most common cause of death, and seizures. It is addictive.

## OTHER SYMPATHOMIMETICS-EPHEDRINE, PSEUDOEPHEDRINE AND PHENYLPROPANOLAMINE

Ephedrine occurs naturally in the plant genus Ephedra and has been a component of ancient Chinese medicine for many centuries. This, and other herbal sources of stimulants, has been reviewed recently by Bucci. Pseudoephedrine and phyenylpropanolamine are synthetic drugs.

This group of drugs are structurally related to amphetamine. Each of the drugs exert their effect indirectly on neurones of the sympathetic and central nervous systems, by displacing noradrenaline and possibly other monoamine transmitters from neuronal storage sites. Both drugs also exert direct effects on adrenergic α and β receptors and are weak inhibitors of monoamine uptake.

They are also resistant to oxidation by the enzyme monoamine oxidase. Both phenylpropanolamine and ephedrine are reported to be 5 times less potent than amphetamine. Pseudoephedrine is reported to be 20 times less potent than ephedrine at least in terms of its cardiovascular actions. The CNS effects of phenylpropanolamine and ephedrine are also much less than those of amphetamine. For example a 75 mg/70 kg body weight dose of ephedrine is required before it will cross the blood-brain barrier. This may explain why both drugs produce much less depletion of brain monoamines than amphetamine.

The effects of phenylpropanolamine and the ephedrines are produced within 40 minutes after administration and can last up to 3 hours with therapeutic effects being associated with plasma levels of between 60 and 200 mg/ml. Both phenylpropanolamine and ephedrine were sold in pharmacies in the UK and USA as constituents of 'cold cures' but phenylpropanolamine has now been proscribed by the US authorities.

### Adverse Effects

At the usual therapeutic doses quoted previously the most common side-effects are tachycardia, hypertension, headache and dizziness. Phenylpropanolamine appears to produce serious hypertensive side-effects at doses sometimes as low as 25 mg. These drugs may cause anorexia, insomnia, irritability and nervousness at low to medium doses, whereas high doses are associated with mania and a psychosis similar to that occasionally seen with amphetamine.

## ABUSE IN SPORT

Abuse of ephedrine, pseudoephedrine and phenylpropanolamine by athletes is nebulous since many of those detected as having taken them have claimed they were using the drugs as 'cold cures'.

The first comprehensive study of the possible ergogenic effects of these drugs was carried out by Sidney and Lefcoe. They examined the effect of 25 mg of ephedrine versus placebo in a double-blind crossover study using three separate athletic trials during a 3-week period. In this comprehensive experiment 10 variables were measured including strength, endurance, reaction time, anaerobic capacity and speed of recovery from effort.

The results showed that, though exercise heart rate and resting pulse pressure increased and post-exercise recovery rate slowed, none of the physical performance measures improved. It was also interesting that no subjective improvements in performance were noted. Using phenylpropanolamine, Swain found no effect on VO2max or perceived exertion compared with placebo.

Further evidence that ephedrine is positively ergogenic is contradictory. In South Africa, found that 120 mg of pseudoephedrine had no effect on prolonged exercise, i.e. a 40 km time-trial 'ride' on a cycle ergometer, or on skeletal muscle function during the ride. By contrast, Bell's group in Canada measured the effects of 120 mg of the most potent isomer, ephedrine, on power output (electrically braked ergometer) and oxygen debt and VO2max in 16 healthy volunteers. They found that compared with placebo, ephedrine significantly increased power output during the first 10 seconds of cycle exercise but had no effect after this time. Ephedrine also had no effect on O2 deficit or accumulated VO2. Interestingly, caffeine alone had no effect on initial power output but had an additive effect to ephedrine in the first 10 seconds of the test. Ephedrine treatment has been associated with increased plasma glucose levels both before and after exercise and increased plasma lactate and noradrenaline levels after exercise.

Using a pseudoephedrine dose of 1 mg/kg, Swain found no effect on VO2max or exertion in 10 subjects exercising on a bicycle ergometer compared with placebo. While Gill found that pseudoephedrine produced minor increases in maximum torque, peak power and lung function in 22 male volunteers undergoing cycle ergometer tests, it had no effect in the same volunteers when they underwent strength-tests. There is evidence that ephedrine and phenylpropanolamine may become abused as anorexic agents by gymnasts and possibly also by body builders.

## Adverse Effects in Athletes

The adverse effects observed in athletes are similar to those seen in the general population. Recent investigations into potential side-effects of phenylpropanolamine and ephedrine in athletes have centred on the cardiovascular system. Swain found that phenylpropanolamine had no effect on systolic or diastolic blood pressure at a dose of 0.33 or 0.66 mg/kg. At a dose of 1 mg/kg psuedoephedrine increased peak systolic but not diastolic blood pressure, while a 2 mg/kg dose had no effect at all. However, a number of investigators have warned of possible interactions between phenylpropanolamine and ephedrine and non-steroidal anti-inflammatory agents (NSAIDs).

The pharmacology of these anti-inflammatory drugs and it will be seen that they inhibit the production of endogenous vasodilators, the prostaglandins. Since many athletes may take these anti-inflammatory drugs, an interaction leading to a larger than expected rise in blood pressure may occur when NSAIDs and phenylpropanolamine and ephedrine are taken together. Another possible dangerous interaction may occur with phenylpropanolamine and ephedrine taken with caffeine.

## Can Abuse be Justified?

The prescription of ephedrine and phenylpropanolamine-like drugs has been criticized. In the 1972 Olympics, US swimmer, De Mont, was disqualified because of the presence of ephedrine in his urine, which he admitted originated from a medicine.

At Seoul, in 1988, the eventual 100 m silver medallist Linford Christie narrowly escaped disqualification when small traces of 'a cold cure substance' were found in his urine. It has been suggested that phenylpropanolamine and ephedrine may indicate more serious abuse of substances like amphetamine and that their presence is a sign of weaning-off from or a mask for the more powerful drug.

## Cocaine

Cocaine first became available commercially in the 1880s. It was an ingredient of the famous Vin Mariani beloved by Pope Leo XIII, which was named 'the wine for athletes'. Sigmund Freud took the drug to try and cure his own bouts of depression and suggested it as a 'cure all' for others. He exclaimed 'I took for the first time 0.05 gm of cocaine and a few moments later I experienced a sudden exhilaration and a feeling of ease'. The drug fell out of medical use by the 1920s, and social use ten years later, only to reappear in the 1960s as a major drug of abuse.

## Pharmacology

Cocaine affects the brain in a complex way. The most obvious initial effects are a decrease in fatigue, an increase in motor activity and an increase in talkativeness, coupled with a general feeling of euphoria and well-being. These mood changes soon subside and are replaced by a dysphoria (mood lowering). Cocaine is possibly the most addictive agent known.

The mechanism by which cocaine produces these effects is not known fully. Animal studies show that cocaine is a powerful 'reinforcer' and rewarding agent. It stimulates elements of the brain's pleasure and reward 'centres' which are distributed throughout the limbic system of the brain and include the dopamine-rich mesocortical and mesolimbic systems. Much of the reinforcing and rewarding behaviour induced by cocaine in animals, i.e. rats, who will repeatedly administer cocaine to themselves in preference to food, can be reduced by dopamine receptor antagonists. The evidence for the action of cocaine on these systems has been reviewed by Fibiger. Further evidence for the involvement of cocaine with dopamine-releasing neurones comes from studies at the molecular level reviewed by Kuhar.

He has shown that cocaine inhibits the re-uptake of dopamine (DA) into the nerve terminals of dopamine-releasing neurones, and it has a similar though less potent effect on noradrenaline uptake in noradenergic neurones. This initially leads to a potentiation of the action of DA at post-synaptic receptor sites. This acute effect of cocaine on the dopamine transporter has been demonstrated by many investigations but it is also exhibited by other drugs, such as methylphenidate, which do not have the same addictive potential as cocaine. In chronic cocaine abusers, in vivo scanning of behaviourally important areas of the cerebral cortex has shown a significant reduction in dopamine D2 receptors associated with decreased dopamine metabolism.

There are also significant decreases in dopamine release in such abusers and these interrelated actions may be part of a mechanism leading to reduced activities of cerebral 'reward circuits' in cocaine abuse and subsequent addiction. However, though dopamine receptor antagonists appear to antagonize all the actions of cocaine in rats, in humans they appear to inhibit cocaine craving, but not the euphoria. Some investigators have linked the dysphoria and craving following a cocaine dose with an increase in post-synaptic receptor numbers though this is contradicted by the studies of Volkow's group. Tricyclic antidepressants which antagonize these post-administration effects are thought to do so by inducing receptor subsensitivity.

Effective treatments for cocaine abuse are still experimental, though a number of potential new cocaine anti-addiction drugs are being investigated. At least two of these have been shown to reduce cocaine self-administration in non-human primates.

### Metabolism

Cocaine is mainly metabolized, by plasma and liver cholinesterases, to benzoyl ecgonine and ecgonine methyl ester, which are excreted in the urine.

## PHARMACOKINETICS

Cocaine may be administered by injection, orally, intranasally or by inhalation. Oral administration produces peak effects at variable times with behavioural changes lasting up to one hour. The most popular route is via nasal 'snorting' which produces peak effects from 5-15 minutes lasting for an hour. Inhalation of 'free-base' cocaine produces peak effects in less than 1 minute, but also a short-lived physiological effect measured in minutes. The route of cocaine administration influences the time course and onset of other actions of cocaine. Effects of the drug such as increases in heart rate and blood pressure are longer lasting via the oral compared with the intravenous route. Smith's group also found that regular cocaine abusers could detect if they were receiving active drug or placebo much quicker via the iv route than the oral and also that iv cocaine is some 10 times more potent than oral cocaine. Inhalation of cocaine results in the most intense cravings compared with other routes of administration. The pharmacological basis for this observation has been determined by Volkow.

They compared levels of dopamine transporter blockade induced by iv, snorted and intranasal cocaine in 32 current cocaine abusers. There was dose-dependent transporter blockade for iv and intranasal delivery but not for smoking. Smoked cocaine produced a self-reported 'high' quicker than the iv route which was quicker than the intranasal route. Differences in the reinforcing effect of cocaine associated with route of administration thus depend not on differences in dopamine transporter blockade but on the speed of entry of cocaine into the brain. The frequency of cocaine administration, at least in rats, also influences the density of brain opioid and dopamine receptors and this needs to be considered in future human research.

## ADVERSE EFFECTS

Cocaine is highly addictive and the abuser may experience acute psychotic symptoms and undertake irrational actions, in addition to the well known adverse effects of euphoria. Chronic symptoms include a paranoid psychosis similar to that induced by amphetamine, coupled with spells of delirium and confusion. Other CNS side-effects include epileptogenesis-that is stimulation of epileptic seizures.

This adverse effect is particularly dangerous since animal studies have revealed that the epileptogenic effect increases with frequency of cocaine abuse, a process known as reverse tolerance which is important when the powerful reinforcing properties of the drug are considered. The epileptogenic effect can be produced even by repeated small doses of the drug which may be more toxic than the same dose given less frequently.

Cocaine abuse is strongly associated with cerebrovascular accidents arising either from the rupture or spasm of cerebral blood vessels. Some of these incidents may be due to pre-existing vascular pathologies, but there are several cases where no predisposing cause has been found at autopsy. Cocaine is also responsible for a number of cardiovascular side-effects, those relating. A recent review of the literature relating to cocaine-induced coronary disease by Benzaquen reveals that a number of factors may influence the development of cardiovascular pathology in cocaine abusers.

Original ideas suggesting a simple mismatch between myocardial oxygen supply and demand caused by cocaine-induced vasoconstriction and the resulting increased myocardial workload are too simplistic. They have argued that a more complex interaction between three key factors: coronary vasoconstriction, intracoronary thrombosis and accelerated atherosclerosis may be involved, as all three can be induced by cocaine abuse. Smith and Perry have suggested that the increase in cardiovascular and cerebrovascular side-effects seen in recent years is due to the rise in abuse of 'crack' cocaine, which is rapidly absorbed and produces a concentrated effect on cerebral arterioles. A detailed account of cocaine side-effects is given by Wadler and Hainline. A summary of the neuropsychiatrie effects of cocaine abuse, including disruption of executive function in prefrontal brain regions is provided by Bolla.

## EFFECTS IN ATHLETES AND ON EXERCISE

Cocaine was used by South American natives for centuries to increase efficiency, vigour and physical endurance. In 1884, Freud tested the effects of 0.1 g of cocaine hydrochloride, taken intranasally, on hand grip strength and on reaction time. He noted that the positive effect of cocaine was greatest when he was fatigued.

In 1930, Theil and Essing reported that 0.1 g of cocaine administered to subjects before exercising on a cycle ergometer improved work efficiency, as determined by VO2 measurements per unit work, and that exercise could be maintained for longer.

The results were attributed to reduced CNS perception of fatigue. A second study using the same cocaine dose revealed no increase in work efficiency but a more rapid increase in recovery after exercise. In his review of pre-1983 studies of the effects of cocaine on exercise, Conlee concluded that they were all contradictory and were usually poorly controlled and carried out. Many of the studies reviewed since 1983 have been in animals because of ethical considerations and have involved measurements undertaken in rats trained to run on treadmills connected to ergometer s.

Early studies have demonstrated that cocaine had no beneficial effect on running times within a dose range of 0.1-20.0 mg/kg bodyweight and at doses above 12.5 mg/kg the cocaine actually reduced running time. At all doses used, cocaine significantly increases glycogen degradation while increasing plasma lactate concentration without producing consistent changes in plasma catecholamine levels. In 1991 Conlee and co-workers demonstrated in rats exercising voluntarily that cocaine increases glycogen metabolism and enhances the exercise-induced sympathetic responses. None of these studies have explained how cocaine reduces endurance performance.

Conlee suggested three possible mechanisms to explain cocaine's action that could operate in parallel:

- Cocaine releases catecholamines which increase glycogenolysis and lactate production leading to early fatigue;
- Cocaine may induce skeletal muscle vasoconstriction, reducing oxygen delivery, oxidative metabolism, strength and reaction time, and stimulating glycogen breakdown; and

- Cocaine may have a direct effect on muscle glycogen breakdown. Indirect evidence originally suggested that mechanism is less likely since cocaine-induced reduction of myocardial bloodflow is not associated with increased myocardial glycogen breakdown, but in 1994, Braiden et al. demonstrated a three-fold increase in muscle lactate accumulation in the white vastus muscle of rats under cocaine-exercise conditions.

These experiments in animals may explain the detrimental effects of cocaine, but do not explain the continued use of the drug and the claims made for it. Perhaps there are other aspects of the action of cocaine which may contribute to the perception that it is ergogenic. Hanna investigated the effects of male coca leaf chewing on exercise/performance in male habitual coca leaf chewers in the Peruvian Andes. He found that compared with non-chewers there was no significant effect of coca chewing on exercise or recovery rates or blood pressure. A further study found that coca leaf chewing did not increase work capacity but might increase endurance times. In these studies cocaine blood levels were not measured and the stated 4.5 g 'dose' of leaves was not strictly regulated.

A more sophisticated study of the effect of coca leaf has been described by Spielvogel. In this experiment, metabolic and hormonal changes in habitual coca chewers were compared with non-coca chewers during incremental exercise to exhaustion. The coca leaf ingestion was controlled at 12 g and this produced a mean cocaine blood concentration of 72 ng/ml. At rest, both habitual and naive coca chewers had similar noradrenaline and adrenaline plasma levels but habitual chewers had higher free fatty acid levels. During exercise, oxygen uptake and work efficiency were similar in both groups, while in incremental exercise habitual chewers demonstrated lower arterial oxygen saturation, which was not due to reduced ventilatory response. Free fatty acid levels were increased during incremental exercise in the coca chewers.

This interesting study remains inconclusive as the possible 'benefits' of raised free fatty acid levels could not be determined. There were no simultaneous measurements of changes in carbohydrate metabolism or endurance. Therefore it is unclear whether a carbohydrate-sparing 'mechanism' was activated by coca chewing and since catecholamine (i.e. noradrenaline and adrenaline) plasma levels remained unaltered, the mechanism for the elevation of plasma free fatty acid was unknown.

A similar increase in free fatty acid concentration following coca chewing has been described by Favier though they observed increased adrenaline and free fatty acid levels during exercise, coupled with lower blood glucose concentrations. Their conclusion was that this might be evidence that cocaine might prolong work and postpone fatigue by increasing fat mobilization and sparing glycogen utilization, but it did not increase time to exhaustion. Thus the previous reviews of this topic still correct in stating that cocaine appears to have no established benefit in exercise/ athletic performance. Longterm cocaine smoking is associated with reduced maximum exercise performance, which is probably due to poor motivation or altered perception

likely since cocaine-induced reduction of myocardial bloodflow is not associated with increased myocardial glycogen breakdown, but in 1994, Braiden et al. demonstrated a three-fold increase in muscle lactate accumulation in the white vastus muscle of rats under cocaine-exercise conditions.

These experiments in animals may explain the detrimental effects of cocaine, but do not explain the continued use of the drug and the claims made for it. Perhaps there are other aspects of the action of cocaine which may contribute to the perception that it is ergogenic. Hanna investigated the effects of male coca leaf chewing on exercise/performance in male habitual coca leaf chewers in the Peruvian Andes.

He found that compared with non-chewers there was no significant effect of coca chewing on exercise or recovery rates or blood pressure. A further study found that coca leaf chewing did not increase work capacity but might increase endurance times. In these studies cocaine blood levels were not measured and the stated 4.5 g 'dose' of leaves was not strictly regulated.

A more sophisticated study of the effect of coca leaf has been described by Spielvogel. In this experiment, metabolic and hormonal changes in habitual coca chewers were compared with non-coca chewers during incremental exercise to exhaustion. The coca leaf ingestion was controlled at 12 g and this produced a mean cocaine blood concentration of 72 ng/ml. At rest, both habitual and naive coca chewers had similar noradrenaline and adrenaline plasma levels but habitual chewers had higher free fatty acid levels.

During exercise, oxygen uptake and work efficiency were similar in both groups, while in incremental exercise habitual chewers demonstrated lower arterial oxygen saturation, which was not due to reduced ventilatory response. Free fatty acid levels were increased during incremental exercise in the coca chewers. This interesting study remains inconclusive as the possible 'benefits' of raised free fatty acid levels could not be determined. There were no simultaneous measurements of changes in carbohydrate metabolism or endurance. Therefore it is unclear whether a carbohydrate-sparing 'mechanism' was activated by coca chewing and since catecholamine (i.e. noradrenaline and adrenaline) plasma levels remained unaltered, the mechanism for the elevation of plasma free fatty acid was unknown.

A similar increase in free fatty acid concentration following coca chewing has been described by Favier though they observed increased adrenaline and free fatty acid levels during exercise, coupled with lower blood glucose concentrations. Their conclusion was that this might be evidence that cocaine might prolong work and postpone fatigue by increasing fat mobilization and sparing glycogen utilization, but it did not increase time to exhaustion. Thus the previous reviews of this topic are still correct in stating that cocaine appears to have no established benefit in exercise/athletic performance.

Longterm cocaine smoking is associated with reduced maximum exercise performance, which is probably due to poor motivation or altered perception of effort. In their critique of the research situation up to 1997, Clarkson and Thompson sympathetically (with regard to ethical issues) analysed the current research by questioning the validity of experiments using coca leaves rather than pure cocaine, even where the plasma cocaine concentration has been subsequently determined. The pharmacokinetics of cocaine may be altered by ingesting it via this route and also the coca leaf may contain other naturally occurring ingredients which might:

- Influence cocaine metabolism and disposition,
- Influence cocaine action at receptors or transporters, and
- Have metabolic effects of their own. Habitual and naive cocaine/coca users may exhibit different responses, and experiments in rats seem to support this. A more detailed analysis of cocaine's effects on exercise in animals has been attempted by Robert Conlee's group since 1995. They demonstrated that cocaine caused an exaggerated rise in the exercise-induced production of lactate and secretion of noradrenaline and adrenaline.

This effect of cocaine on catecholamine secretion could be the basis of the ergolytic effect of cocaine on exercise and may be involved in the response to cocaine in athletes. These cocaine effects may not be caused by a vascular action of noradrenaline since blockade of $\alpha 1$ -receptors does not block the action of cocaine on glycogenolysis or lactic acid production. Since it is quite likely that athletes abusing cocaine will be chronic abusers, Conlee's group compared cocaine responses in naive and chronic cocaine-administered rats. They found that responses to cocaine in terms of noradrenaline and adrenaline release were greater in rats that had previously received cocaine on a regular basis. It may be that cocaine's positive ergogenic effect is manifested only on activities of short duration requiring a burst of high intensity energy output and activities associated with the drug's central stimulatory effect rather than its action on peripheral metabolism. It has been suggested that it is precisely for these central heightened arousal and increased alertness effects, achieved principally at 'low' doses, that cocaine is abused in sport.

A 1984 study quotes 17 per cent of 2039 US NCAA athletes admitting to use cocaine in the year preceding the study. Two years later 50 per cent of the respondents in a survey of US National Football League Players revealed that they felt cocaine was 'the number one drug of abuse in the NFL'. In Chicago, 2.4 per cent of 1117 male high school athletes admitted to using cocaine in a study conducted by Forman. It is not clear from these surveys whether the cocaine was abused for social or athletic performance-enhancing reasons.

## Side-effects in Athletes

In the previous edition of this book a paper detailing the deaths of two athletes from cocaine abuse was described. These sudden deaths of a basketball player and a US footballer from cocaine-induced coronary occlusion provided the most dramatic evidence of the potential adverse side-effects of cocaine abuse in athletes. In this paper, Cantwell and Rose describe the recovery of a 21-year-old cocaine and amphetamine abusing athlete from a coronary occlusion. These cases were followed by the cocaine-related deaths of basketball players Bias and Rogers in 1986.

The authors have also described the reported experiences of several US baseball players who testify to the mood-enhancing but often performance-inhibiting effects of cocaine. Significantly, baseball players complained of the deleterious central effects of cocaine, i.e. they were most liable to misjudge pitching and hitting. The authors also reported time disorientation in basketball players. New York Yankees' pitcher Steve Howe was arraigned on charges of cocaine abuse in 1991, but escaped a lifetime ban from baseball. The apparent leniency of US Baseball League administrators towards drug transgression has been criticized.

There have also been reports of athletes combining cocaine abuse with other drugs such as alcohol and anabolic steroids. According to Welder and Melchert heavy alcohol consumption combined with cocaine abuse enhances cocaine's cardiotoxicity, possibly by the production of a unique metabolite 'cocaethylene'. The existence and structure of cocaethylene, as the ethyl ester of the cocaine metabolite benzoylecgonine, has been established by Farre and its actions in animals and man have been reviewed and investigated by McCance-Katz. They have detailed the following facts: that cocaine and alcohol taken together have additive deleterious effects, that simultaneous consumption of alcohol and cocaine leads to the formation of cocaethylene, and that though cocaethylene is less potent than cocaine, it is eliminated more slowly and could thus accumulate during or following an alcohol/cocaine binge. Further dangers arise from the possibility that the increased sense of well-being produced by the cocaine/alcohol mixture would lead to further abuse leading to increased toxicity from the drugs plus the toxicity of cocaethylene. Is this relevant to sport? Most certainly it is.

This may well have been the ultimate cause of death of the Canadian ice-hockey player John Kordic who abused cocaine, alcohol and anabolic steroids. His downfall has been chronicled in detail by Scher and included frequent fights on the pitch, with opponents, team-mates and officials. 'Whatever sporting advantage might be gained by cocaine abuse is far outweighed by the serious cardiovascular consequences'.

It is quite possible that it is the occasional short-term abuse in sport which is the major problem and athletes think that such an abuse pattern will prevent their experiencing harmful side-effects. However, as with anabolic steroids, the cardiotoxic damage is probably insidious; with any current cardiac damage causing problems in later life. Another aspect is that much of the cocaine abuse in sport may be social, with young, naive individuals, suddenly with massive salaries, able to fund an experimental abuse that leads to addiction.

## CAFFEINE, THEOPHYLLINE AND OTHER METHYL XANTHINES

The three psychoactive drugs most commonly used are alcohols, nicotine and caffeine and all are self-administered! It has been suggested that caffeine has been in use as a stimulant since the Stone Age! Caffeine is a member of the methyl xanthine group of compounds, which also includes theophylline and theobromine. Caffeine occurs naturally in coca, coffee beans and tea leaves. The amount of caffeine obtained from each source depends on the method of extraction and the particle size of the extracts. Caffeine is added to soft drinks such as many types of colas and is also present in a number of 'over-the-counter' medicines.

## Pharmacology

Caffeine usually exerts an effect on the CNS in doses ranging from 85-200 mg and in this dose range it produces a reduction in drowsiness and fatigue, an elevation in mood, improved alertness and productivity, increasing capacity for sustained intellectual effort and a rapid and clearer flow of thought.

**Table:** Caffeine Content of some Beverages, Drinks and Medicines

| *Caffeine content (mg)* | *Coffee (per 5 oz cup)* |
|---|---|
| Percolated | 64-124 |
| Instant | 40-108 |
| Filter | 110-150 |
| Decaffeinated | 2-5 |
| Tea (per 5 oz cup) | |
| 1 minute brew | 9-33 |
| 5 minute brew | 25-50 |
| Soft drinks (per 12 oz serving) | |
| Pepsi Cola | 38.4 |
| Coca-Cola | 46 |
| Proprietary medicines | |
| Anadin tablet | 15 |
| Cephos tablet | 10 |
| Coldrex cold treatment tablet | 25 |
| Phensic tablet | 50 |

This dose range of caffeine also causes diuresis, a relaxation of smooth muscle, activation of gastric acid secretion and an increase in heart rate, blood pressure and blood vessel diameter.

A caffeine dose in excess of 250 mg is considered to be high and may cause headaches, instability and nervousness. The American Psychiatric Association considers caffeine intoxication as occurring at doses greater than 250 mg. The pharmacokinetics of caffeine has been comprehensively reviewed by Sawynok and Yaksh. They concluded that caffeine absorption after oral administration is almost 100 per cent and that caffeine can appear in the blood in as little as 5 min after ingestion. An important point is that though peak plasma concentrations usually occur 30-60 min after oral administration, the range can be as wide as 15-20 min because of individual variations in gastric emptying. Using an oral dose of 175 mg, it can be shown that almost 90 per cent of the caffeine dose can be absorbed from the stomach giving rise to plasma concentrations of 5-10 μg/ml.

In 17 subjects who consumed coffee and tea, with an average daily consumption of 6.8 mg/kg per day of caffeine, mean 24 h plasma levels of 4.4 μg/ml were observed. The range of concentrations during the 24 h sampling period was 1.2-9.7 μg/ml. This information has important consequences for athletes who drink caffeine-containing beverages regularly and who might take additional pure caffeine, as the plasma levels of the two ingestions will be additive. They should also be aware that caffeine is absorbed more slowly from soft drinks such as Coca-Cola than from tea or coffee. Caffeine is water and lipid soluble and is therefore rapidly distributed through all tissues from the plasma and moves into the brain rapidly by simple diffusion. The plasma half-life, that is the time for a given concentration in the plasma to reduce by half, varies from 3-5 hours. Five important features governing caffeine disposition relevant to athletes.

These are age, genetics, exercise, smoking and other drugs. Caffeine, like all methyxanthines, is metabolized by the liver P450 enzyme system to theophylline (4 per cent), theobromine (12 per cent) and paraxanthine (84 per cent). This system also metabolizes the hydrocarbons produced by tobacco smoke, and several common drugs such as the phenobarbitone, the new serotonin-selective re-uptake inhibitor (SSRI) antidepressants and the steroids of oral contraceptives. This has been reviewed recently by Sinclair and Geiger. Several studies have shown that age has very little effect on caffeine metabolism, but there can be marked genetic variabilities in the ability to metabolize it.

Moderate exercise appears to increase peak plasma concentrations of caffeine. Smoking increases caffeine removal from the plasma, by increasing the rate at which it is metabolized. Drugs as varied as oral contraceptives, the SSRI antidepressants and alcohol reduce caffeine metabolism, thus raising its plasma levels. Strenuous exercise decreases caffeine elimination more in women than in men.

Some researchers have suggested the optimum ergogenic effect of caffeine occurs 3 hours after ingestion, which correlates with an apparent peak in lipolysis. This theory has been discounted by Graham as there is no evidence that the increased lipolysis correlates with ergogenicity. Many athletes are convinced that caffeine improves their performance, while many a student have improved their mental concentration by taking drinks containing caffeine. These uses aside, it must be remembered that caffeine consumption (as coffee) has been associated with a number of systemic disorders which include hypertension, myocardial infarction, peptic ulcer and cancers of the gastrointestinal tract and urinary tract.

An interesting study by Graham showed that caffeine contained in normal coffee was much less effective in improving the endurance of athletes in a 10 km run than equivalent doses of pure caffeine. Later Graham compared this result with other studies which indicated that coffee was an ergogenic aid. He concluded that coffee may also contain compounds with an anti-ergogenic effect. This should be considered in further studies as should the possible confounding of any results by smoking, since tobacco hydrocarbons alter the activity of enzymes that metabolize caffeine.

There have been suggestions that combination of caffeine with carbohydrate supplements enhances the ergogenicity of both substances compared to when either is used alone. Graham found the evidence for this inconclusive but did conclude that there was no detrimental effect with a combination of caffeine and carbohydrate supplements.

## The Effects of Caffeine

*Caffeine causes:*

- Increased gastric acid and pepsin secretion plus increased secretion into the small intestine;
- Increased heart rate, stroke volume, cardiac output and blood pressure at rest;
- Tachycardia;
- Increased lipolysis;
- Increased contractility of skeletal muscles;
- Increased oxygen consumption and metabolic rate;
- Increased diuresis;
- Increased anti-nociceptive action of NSAIDs and exerts a mild antinociceptive action itself.

## Mechanism of Action

Caffeine is a powerful inhibitor of the cyclic nucleotide phosphodiesterase group of enzymes, of which there are five distinct types. These enzymes inactivate the so-called intracellular 'second messengers', such as cyclic AMP, which act as one of the links between receptor stimulation and cellular response. When these cellular enzymes are inhibited the action of intracellular messengers such as cyclic AMP is increased. For many years, researchers doubted that this was the main mechanism of action of caffeine since the intracellular concentration of caffeine (0.1-1 mmol) required to achieve significant enzyme inhibition could not be produced by the blood concentrations provided by normal caffeine dosing.

However, phosphodiesterase inhibition as a mechanism of action should not be entirely dismissed. Caffeine also inhibits 52 -nucleotidase enzymes which convert AMP to adenosine, but this has not been thought to be of consequence in the mechanism of action of caffeine. However, recent research by Latini and Perdata suggests that this action may need to be investigated owing to the possible role of adenosine as a tissue mediator during tissue ischaemia.

It is now widely accepted that the majority of the pharmacological effects of caffeine are mediated by antagonism of adenosine receptors, though some of the cardiac and renal actions may still be brought about by inhibition of phosphodiesterases. In 1983, Daly et al. showed that the central stimulatory activity of caffeine is correlated with its ability to bind to and inhibit adenosine receptors. There are currently four types of adenosine receptor (A1, A2A, A2B and A3) and the relative importance of these is still under investigation.

Reviews of current literature by Nyce and Sinclair and Geiger the widespread distribution and complex actions of the adenosine receptor sub-types. Activation of receptors depresses neurotransmission, induces sleep, suppresses pain, causes bronchoconstriction and sodium retention and opposes the action of β receptors. Stimulation of A2 receptors leads to peripheral and cerebral vasodilatation and inhibition of inflammation, while A3 receptor stimulation inactivates eosinophil migration.

An intriguing insight into the significance of adenosine receptors in metabolism and exercise is revealed by Latini and Perdata. They state that the higher affinity A, and A2A adenosine receptors are those involved in 'normal' adenosine neurotransmission. Under conditions of increased metabolic activity or a mismatch between energy supply and demand, adenosine is released from non-neuronal cells (possibly tissue mediators) and this extra adenosine is sufficient to stimulate the less sensitive A3 receptors. Since caffeine is a weak antagonist of these A3 receptors, this may be a mechanism by which caffeine produces some of its effects. It is also apparent that caffeine and other methyl xanthines may influence the response to ischaemia during exercise, since adenosine acting on A1 and A3 receptors may have a pre-conditioning and protective effect towards ischaemia in cardiac and striated muscle. Since caffeine, theobromine and theophylline are potent antagonists of A, and A2 receptors, and caffeine is a weak antagonist of A3 receptors, it can be seen that the actions of caffeine on individuals either at rest or during exercise will take some time to evaluate fully. Central effects.

Caffeine is widely accepted as a mild stimulant, though clinical tests often reveal a wide variability in its action. Caffeine increases vigilance, attention and prevents the decrement in performance and information processing that occurs during fatigue or where boring repetitive jobs are being carried out. Compared with controls, subjects taking caffeine report improved alertness, reaction times and attention span.

The common finding of most placebo-controlled studies carried out in the last 30 years is that caffeine produces the most consistent improvements in tests where fatigue or a stressful workload are part of the research protocol. Investigations into the effects of caffeine on numerical reasoning, verbal fluency, short-term memory or digital skill have produced conflicting results. This may be explained by the effect of differences in personality on the action of caffeine; that is, extroverts may react differently to introverts. The impulsiveness of subjects may also influence their response to caffeine, as may their normal pattern of caffeine consumption.

Many subjects report increased feelings of well-being indicated by improvements in mood, vigour and euphoria. However, some researchers have shown that the response to caffeine is dependent on expectations and that in controlled trials subjects are able to detect caffeine from placebo. The most favourable improvements in mood seem to occur when doses of up to 100-200 mg are taken.

When the dose exceeds 400 mg the major response seems to be dysphoria (lowering of mood) and increased anxiety. It has been suggested that caffeine may act as a reinforcing agent in that caffeine abstinence for up to 24 h following chronic caffeine consumption leads to a withdrawal state characterized by irritability, insomnia, muscle twitching and headaches. Avoidance of this negative state could therefore act as a reinforcement of caffeine administration. Tolerance to and dependency on caffeine have been described by Strain and Griffins who state that such dependent individuals exhibit all the symptoms characteristic of substance dependency. Tolerance has been claimed to be associated with an up-regulation of adenosine A1 or A2 receptors, but this may not occur in humans.

Caffeine has been shown to be anxiogenic in a number of studies and this has led to the description of a clinical syndrome-caffeinism-by Greden. The anxiogenic or alerting effect may be caused by antagonism by caffeine of adenosine action at CNS A2 receptors, where adenosine has a sedative effect. This 'alerting' action of caffeine may well be coupled to the reduction in 'perceived exertion' measurable in inactive and exercising volunteers whereby athletes feel they have done less work and expended less energy than they actually have.

## Adverse Reactions

When coffee drinking became fashionable in Great Britain during the seventeenth century the effects of caffeine were immediately noticed and there were suggestions that it should be banned.

The average intake of caffeine in the USA is 206 mg per person per day and 10 per cent of the population consume greater than 1000 mg per day. The major side-effects have been described and categorized as acute, severe and chronic by Wadler and Hainline. Mild effects include nervousness, irritability, insomnia and gastrointestinal distress.

Severe effects include peptic ulcer, delirium, coma, seizures and supraventricular and ventricular arrhythmias, associated with doses greater than 200 mg/kg. Chronic effects mainly involve raised serum cholesterol levels. A particular cluster of side-effects involving anxiety, mood changes, sleep disruption, psychophysiological changes and withdrawal symptoms has been recognized as caffeinism and is described by Greden. The Diagnostic and Statistical Manual of Mental Disorders (DSM IV) of the American Psychiatric Association describes caffeine intoxication as a condition simulating an anxiety attack in which the person experiences nausea, insomnia, restlessness and jitteriness.

## EFFECTS IN ATHLETES

In 1965 Bellet et al. described the elevation of blood fatty acids that occurred with caffeine ingestion. They concluded that caffeine improved endurance by enhancing fat utilization, thus sparing glycogen stores.

Using nine competitive cyclists, Costill studied the effects of caffeine on their general metabolism. Each cyclist exercised to exhaustion on a cycle ergometer at 50 per cent of their aerobic capacity after ingesting either decaffeinated or normal coffee (containing 330 mg caffeine). The caffeine takers managed to exercise for 19.5 per cent longer than the control group and had significantly higher levels of plasma fatty acids and blood glycerol. In the caffeine group, the respiratory quotient (RQ) was reduced, possibly indicating a shift from carbohydrate to fat utilization. It was suggested that increased lipolysis postponed exhaustion by slowing the rate of glycogen utilization in liver and skeletal muscle. Ivy et al. found that caffeine increased work production in athletes by 7.4 per cent compared with control conditions and in the same study fat oxidation was elevated by 31 per cent during the last 70 min of the trial.

Essig measured the effect of caffeine on insulin secretion and glycogen utilization in seven untrained male cyclists. Compared with controls, the caffeine group had a 51 per cent increase in lipid oxidation. Muscle biopsies showed a 39 per cent reduction in glycogen utilization. They concluded that caffeine ingestion can increase oxidation of fatty acids and glycerol in muscle. In contrast, Perkins and Williams could find no effect with 4, 7 or 10 mg of caffeine per kg body weight in 14 male students exercising to exhaustion. They found no significant difference between control and caffeine-taking groups in exercise time to exhaustion, even though there was a caffeine-induced increase in fatty acid level. In the 6 years since the last edition of this book, the glycogen sparing theory has not advanced further.

Two studies in 2000 by Laurent and Graha failed to demonstrate any glycogen sparing at 60 and 70 per cent VO2max, respectively. Many of these older studies, though often well-controlled, did not measure the substances about which they were speculating! Several studies have indicated a role for lactate in the mechanism of action of caffeine as it has been shown to raise blood lactate levels. Graham et al. compared the effect of caffeine administration with placebo in individuals where one leg was exercised while the other was static. Arterial lactate levels rose in the caffeine-treated subjects compared with placebo, but lactate exchange was unaltered by caffeine in either the exercising or the non-exercising leg. The role of lactate is thus unclear.

The results of the pioneering studies of the putative ergogenicity of caffeine led me to summarize in the previous editions of this book that 'caffeine has a positive ergogenic effect on large muscles and on short term exercise which requires both strength and power'.

Since then a number of studies have been carried out in both animals and humans, some of which support and some of which refute this statement. By the 1990s some reviewers began to have doubts whether caffeine was a true ergogenic aid. In his 1991 review, Conlee listed six crucial factors which he claimed accounted for the variability in the effect of caffeine on athletic performance.

These were dose, type of exercise, intensity of exercise, pre-exercise feedings, previous caffeine use and training status. He also identified from his literature survey optimal conditions for the ergogenic effect of caffeine, which are: use of untrained, caffeine-abstaining subjects, caffeine doses of 6-10 mg/kg, abstinence from high carbohydrate diets and an experimental protocol involving prolonged activities at 70-85 per cent VO2max. Some of the questions raised by Conlee had also been addressed previously by Powers and Dodd, who reviewed the evidence for caffeine ergogenicity prior to 1985 and in particular noted discrepancies between the positive effect of caffeine during graded exercise but its lack of effect on VO2max.

Research evidence has been further complicated by the increasing number of animal studies, particularly those involving isolated muscle preparations. A detailed analysis of the conflicting results produced by these various studies was made by Dodd. They examined all the studies of caffeine on exercise performance and found that they could be divided into three major groups, including short-term high-intensity exercise, graded incremental exercise and prolonged endurance exercise, each group containing both human and animal studies.

During short-term high-intensity exercise, caffeine was shown to enhance muscle force production in isolated muscle preparations while most human studies demonstrate no effect. Caffeine appears to increase peak muscular tension and decrease the time required to achieve peak tension and this is associated with increased release of $Ca^{2+}$ from the sarcoplasmic reticulum. However, in this situation, the muscle $Ca^{2+}$ was also depleted more rapidly resulting in earlier fatigue. Studies in humans, however, have shown that caffeine does not increase force, electromyographic activity or muscular power during either hand grip exercise or short maximal bouts of cycle exercise. Dodd have concluded that the major source of discrepancy between human and in vitro animal studies is the dosage of caffeine used.

They have calculated that most in vitro studies utilize caffeine doses of 200-3500 μmol/1, while human studies have used caffeine doses below 10 mg/kg. In the blood, even assuming the caffeine remained unbound to plasma proteins, the concentration of caffeine would be 60-100 μmol/l. If the allowance is made for 15-17 per cent binding of caffeine to plasma proteins then the amount of caffeine available for cellular action is some 100 μmol less than the lowest dosage used in in vitro studies. Conversely, to produce a positive ergogenic effect in humans of the same order as that achieved during in vitro experiments, it would require caffeine doses which would produce urinary caffeine concentrations well in excess of the ICO limits of 12 μg/ml urine. It is surprising that so few caffeine studies have involved determinations of blood caffeine levels following administration and during exercise.

More recently, the effects of caffeine on graded incremental exercise have been investigated. Two studies, both of which administered caffeine at 10-15 mg/kg to moderately fit, caffeine-naive subjects, 1-3 hours before exercise testing, demonstrated an improved performance during graded incremental exercise. Performance improvement was identified as an increase in time to exhaustion, and a reduced lactate threshold. The significance of the results is that they were obtained using high doses of caffeine and it is unclear whether they were influenced by any caffeine intolerance of the subjects. However, in 1993, Dodd and co-workers produced evidence to show that the caffeine tolerance within a subject has no effect on performance during exercise of moderate intensity and duration. From these findings it was concluded that the results of the original studies were associated with the high dosage of caffeine used.

The other major area of exercise research involving caffeine concerns prolonged endurance exercise, the subject of the much quoted early research of Costill the past four years the initial findings have been disputed. Conlee has stated that the evidence supporting the positive ergogenic effect of caffeine during prolonged exercise is inconclusive. In contrast Dodd have reviewed the studies of caffeine and prolonged exercise since 1978 and have produced a detailed re-analysis of the series of tests. There was a considerable variability in the experimental design used. For example, some studies used caffeine-naive, others caffeinehabituated subjects and dietary control was employed in some subjects but not in others. With the exception of one study that involved a 21 km ski run, all the studies quoted involved cycle ergometer or treadmill measurements.

From these, Dodd concluded that moderate to high doses of caffeine are ergogenic during prolonged moderate-intensity exercise in both caffeine-naive and caffeine-habituated subjects. It was argued in their review that the positive ergogenic effect of caffeine on endurance exercise is apparent only when studies of high intensity exercise are omitted from the analysis. Thus, in their table of endurance studies, two of which used continuous low-intensity exercise (50-60 per cent of VO2max) for 2-8 hours followed by exercise to exhaustion at 90 per cent of VO2max, there was no evidence of an ergogenic effect of caffeine. The biochemical and physiological basis of the ergogenic effect of caffeine during endurance exercise is unclear. The possible explanations cited by Ivy and Essig have been added to by Conlee and now include:

- A stimulatory effect on the CNS,
- Enhanced release of catecholamines,
- Free fatty acid mobilization from adipose tissue leading to increased
- Oxidation in muscle and the sparing of glycogen,
- Indirect inhibition of muscle glycogenolysis, thus sparing muscle glycogen, and
- Increased use of muscle triglycerides, also leading to muscle glycogen sparing.

Studies where caffeine effects on glycogen depletion have been investigated simultaneously with prolonged exercise all show that caffeine brings about glycogen sparing, thus confirming the original hypothesis of Bellet quoted earlier. Research by Essig suggesting that fat metabolism, fuelled by increased lipolysis, is enhanced following caffeine ingestion has not been unequivocally supported by recent research. Dodd quote the results of seven experiments, five of which demonstrate an increase in plasma free fatty acid levels during exercise following caffeine ingestion which, however, was not accompanied in any study by a rise in the respiratory quotient.

Thus caffeine may well antagonize adenosine-mediated inhibition of lipolysis, but the consequent increased availability of free fatty acids does not appear to influence energy production. The anomalous results obtained with caffeine on free fatty acids and the respiratory quotient may be explained by the observation that caffeine ingestion raises plasma catecholamine levels. This may lead to a pre-exercise increase in free fatty acid utilization, which masks any effect of caffeine during the exercise period.

However,that caffeine ingestion immediately prior to exercise to exhaustion improved the distance that was run by six trained athletes. In this experiment blood lactate was raised only at the end of the study and blood triglycerides were elevated by caffeine only after 45 min of exercise. This, then, is the position up to the mid-1990s. In the past 6 years, research into the effects of caffeine has been more intensive, but though we have much further evidence that caffeine is ergogenic, the nature, mechanism and circumstances of its effects in exercise are hardly any clearer. Research has been clouded by investigations into whether the IOC limit of 12 μg/ml urinary concentration is acceptable and also by experiments involving the addition of caffeine to other ergogenic agents and the effects of caffeine added to so-called power supplements. Spriet is adamant that caffeine does have a measurable ergogenic effect on endurance exercise at doses which do not contravene the IOC urinary concentration limit.

Many of the effects of stimulants on exercise are subtle and may only be revealed using the most accurate ergometers and timing devices currently available. There is also confusion about which environment is best to research and observe the effects of caffeine: the controlled laboratory situation or the semi-controlled competitive arena. Terry Graham has attempted to organize the current state of our knowledge about caffeine in a comprehensive review. He has divided caffeine effects into five major categories:

- Endurance in long-term exercise;
- Speed and power in long-term exercise;
- Endurance in short-term intensive exercise;
- Power in short-term intensive exercise; and
- Strength activity.

Comparing results over the past 6 years and back to 1981, he found 13 studies which examined the effect of caffeine on endurance exercise and only two failed to find a positive ergogenic effect for caffeine. In these experiments, power was kept constant or controlled so that the only 'athletic' variable being measured was endurance time. His review concludes that whether this is a true increase of the competition situation is debatable but that, even so, such an effect of caffeine might be useful in training.

The earlier studies on speed and power have often been criticized for the small numbers of subjects involved and the lack of vigour in the protocol design. Power and speed studies tend to be more equivocal but still seem, on balance, to support an ergogenic effect of caffeine. In contrast to the highly positive effect of caffeine on speed in cross-country skiers, Cole showed that caffeine ingestion did not benefit one athlete in a 21 km road run. Caffeine reduced the 1.5 km time by 23 seconds in a group of 12 swimmers. In a well-controlled study by Kovacs caffeine enhanced the power output by 20 cyclists in a 1 hour time-trial, but this study was complicated by the co-administration of a power/electrolyte drink: the effects of caffeine being additive.

## Short-term Endurance and Internal Exercise

Collomp and his group found no effect of caffeine on exercise duration at VO2max compared with placebo, while Jackman's groupn found there was a statistically significant effect of caffeine on endurance under these conditions. Analysis of five studies of caffeine in progressive exercise regimes has shown that in four of these, caffeine or theophylline has a positive effect, or at least 'a non-significant improvement in exercise time'. Pasman found that though incremental doses of caffeine enhanced endurance performance time in cyclists exercising to exhaustion on an ergometer, there was no dose-response relationship between caffeine and performance or blood glycerol concentration.

During short-term intensive exercise the effects of caffeine seem to be more equivocal. We now seem to be in a position to overturn the perceived wisdom that caffeine has no effects on power output in these conditions. Whereas Wiles' group in 1992 showed that caffeine improved running speed in non-elite athletes, the degree of improvement did not correlate with caffeine intake. Collomp's group of four trained swimmers improved their 100 m sprint times while taking caffeine, whereas a group of untrained swimmers noted no improvement.

Thus, caffeine does seem to have an ergogenic effect in at least four categories of exercise evaluation. How is this achieved? Early experiments rely heavily on the so-called 'glycogen-sparing theory': caffeine stimulates adrenaline secretion resulting in increased lipolysis and plasma free fatty acid (FFA) concentration, increased fat oxidation and a reduction in the utilization of carbohydrate. Graham has stated that there is now much less support for this hypothesis, particularly since caffeine has now been shown to enhance aspects of short-term and/or intense activity exercise in which the influence of fatty acids is negligible.

Also, van Baak and Saris have demonstrated that FFAs are not elevated in the blood during endurance performance exercise regimes. He has revised the theory: caffeine stimulates FFA release by antagonizing A1 adenosine receptors on adipocytes, increased FFA concentration is taken up by the liver, which oxidizes them or converts them to triglycerides. Excess FFAs are partially oxidized to keto acids (ketone bodies), which can be used as an energy source by muscle, heart and other tissues. Central to the older hypotheses is the concept of glycogen sparing.

Chesley found no difference in the glycogen content of exercising muscle either 3 or 15 minutes into an exercise regime at 85 per cent of VO2max and Greer have shown that theophylline and caffeine increased endurance time, but did not change muscle glycogen depletion. Further work needs to be done to investigate these conflicts, possibly re-evaluating and re-running the earlier experiments. Graham has cited six reports of caffeine-induced increases in blood glucose but states that generally it has little or no effect. To add to the confusion surrounding caffeine action, it has frequently been demonstrated in the past that it increases blood lactate levels during exercise. However, this increase in lactate does not originate from the muscle, as demonstrated recently by Graham's team, and they were able to demonstrate no effect of caffeine or theophylline on fat or carbohydrate metabolism during exercise.

Recent work by Chesley concluded that caffeine may reduce phosphocreatine degradation and reduce the formation of ADP in exercising muscle, but this was carried out in a small sample of volunteers. Caffeine increases plasma adrenaline levels, but this increase does not seem to be related to caffeine-induced improvements in endurance, power output or speed during exercise. One recent study has demonstrated a caffeine-induced increase in noradrenaline release in exercising muscle and this needs to be investigated in relation to different exercise programmes in a concentration- and dose-dependent manner. So, if we have destroyed the fashionable glycogen/lactate/FFA theories; what remains?

Other possibilities for caffeine mechanisms of action include: actions on ion balance, blood flow and the striated muscle excitationcontraction coupling mechanism. The role of adenosine and, therefore, the action of adenosine receptor antagonism in these processes needs to be examined. Another neglected area of caffeine/methyl xanthine research includes the CNS. Each of the adenosine receptor types found in the brain and the full implications for the inhibitor of these receptors on behaviour needs to be investigated. In 1996, Cole et al. showed that caffeine may alter the perception by an athlete of how much exercise they had actually performed. The basis of this may well be simiar to the observations of Plaskett and Cafarelli who showed that alterations in muscle proprioception may be involved in the caffeine-enhanced ability to endure repeated isometric quadriceps contractions. Anselme noted that caffeine enhanced maximum power in 6-second sprints but failed to do so in a 30-second Wingate test.

Graham concluded from this limited evidence that 'caffeine can be ergogenic in exercise lasting as long as 60 seconds'. In this review, Graham notes the many anecdotal reports of caffeine use in strength athletes and suggests that the use could be related to perceived improvements in strength, power or fatigue. His review of the small number of experiments on the direct effects of caffeine on muscle contractility and the spinal reflex also suggests that caffeine may have direct actions on muscle strength, which are disassociated from its assumed metabolic actions. Some support for this theory comes from a small study by Tarnopolsky and Cupido.

They found that caffeine potentiates low frequency (20 Hz) muscle force but has no effect at 40 Hz. This study involved only six volunteers in each of a habitual and non-habitual caffeine group. It may indicate that some of the ergogenic effect of caffeine is produced by a direct effect on muscle. Another largely unresearched area, surprisingly, is in team sports. Paton examined the effect of caffeine on mean sprint performance and fatigue over 10 sprints and found that the effect of caffeine was negligible, and further doses of caffeine worsened the time taken to complete the final sprint compared with placebo.

## CAFFEINE COMBINATIONS

Caffeine appears to have an additive effect on performance when combined with stimulants such as ephedrine. Bell's group in Toronto, Canada have examined the effects of caffeine and ephedrine together in a number of exercise situations. They found that combined caffeine and ephedrine significantly improved performance in the so-called 'harrier test' and resulted in improved run times and increased heart-rate. Using an anaerobic exercise programme found that ephedrine increased power output during the early phase of the test but caffeine increased time to exhaustion. They explained their result on the basis of central stimulation by ephedrine and muscle stimulation by caffeine.

I observed in 1996 that future research might be devoted to understanding the underlying psychological processes that influence the abuse of central stimulants by athletes and possibly those mental factors that contribute to success or failure in sport. Begel in 1992 reviewed the psychodynamic factors influencing the development of the athlete and the maintenance of his/her performance. Several sport scientists have attempted to devise models and measurement techniques for the evaluation of mental and psychological influences on sport. John Raglin's recent review of the MHM revealed that successful athletes enjoyed better mental health than their less successful colleagues and that successful athletes were less likely to be introverted.

He also admitted that mental health in the unsuccessful athletes was still normal when compared with the rest of the population and that introversion has been shown to be advantageous in sports involving extreme manual skill such as shooting. Mood state in many of the studies reviewed by Raglin was closely related to training levels and in particular to overtraining. There may be a connection, then, between reduced performance, overtraining and lowered mood. Possibly, athletes particularly resort to central stimulants when coaches fail to identify or help to rectify problems in the athletes' approach and technique or fail to counsel them adequately when their performance drops.

It would also be interesting to know, as Begel concluded, what particular personalities are associated with central stimulant abuse in sportspersons and whether psychiatric disorders contribute to abuse of stimulants by them. Could there be a biochemical-psychopharmacological connection? The authors of two reviews on the influence of CNS neurotransmission systems on mental and physical performance suggest this is possible. Strüder and Weicker argue that exhaustive, intensive exercise may lead to disruption of normal neurotransmission patterns in the brain, particularly those involving the neurotransmitter 5HT (serotonin).

Their second proposition is that the mental symptoms experienced by many over-training athletes are not caused by systemic metabolic changes but by 'central, exhaustive exercise stress'. It may be too simplistic to link stimulant abuse in sport to tenuous changes in CNS neurotransmission, but since many of the drugs of abuse profound changes in these processes, it is a subject worthy of further investigation. It is interesting that both voluntary running and cocaine administration have similar effects on certain brain 'reward' centres in rats' brains. Perhaps scanning studies will reveal similar findings in the human brain.

## CONCLUSIONS AND THE FUTURE

The effect of stimulants on sporting performance is proving to be more subtle than was originally forecast. Not only are we to revise our concepts of what aspects of performance are enhanced by these drugs but we are having to revisit long-held theories about modes of action. Many of the current anomalies in the results obtained with stimulant drugs could be resolved by more carefully standardized and controlled experiments.

For example, we need to differentiate studies on endurance from speed, power from work and to include analysis of subtle central actions like the perception of work done. It is also obvious that we must control for the subjects' athletic prowess and state of training because this has confounded investigations into anabolic steroids for many years. Studies also illustrate differences in responses between naive and habitual 'users' of a drug in both animal and human studies and this also must be incorporated into experimental design. Finally, we must learn to be more thorough and rigorous in the overall design of our experiments.

Good studies should measure the plasma/blood concentration of any drug being administered together with physiological and physical measures of its effect. Also a full and detailed analysis of the impact of the drug under investigation over time in several exercise paradigms should be undertaken as the maximum effect of ephedrine, for example, seems to occur after only 10 seconds of exercise.

# Chapter 4

# Respiratory Tract Disorder Medicines

Maximum performance in aerobic events, at whatever level of competition, is only achievable if respiratory function is optimal. Participants will always be concerned about respiratory problems, be they major disease such as asthma or minor ailment such as the common cold.

Their recourse to medications either to control or to alleviate symptoms of these conditions has brought many sportspersons into conflict with their national federations and Olympic committees. Thus in the XXVII Olympiad in Sydney, there were 31 positive drug tests reported to the Chairman of the IOC Medical Commission by the head of the Australian Sport Drug Testing Laboratory. Of those 31, 6 were quality control samples.

Of the remaining 25 positive results, 14 were for drugs used to treat asthma and 1 was for treatment of the common cold. No further action was taken against the users of the anti-asthma medications because they were permitted drugs, the quantity used fell within the stipulated urine concentration and prior notification had been provided. However, the drug used to treat the common cold resulted in the loss of a gold medal for the individual concerned.

That drugs used to treat respiratory problems are still of concern to both participants and those responsible for drug testing. The pathophysiology of asthma, exercise-induced asthma and of coughs and colds. The treatments of those conditions with reference to current British Thoracic Society

(BTS) guidelines and to the IOC Regulations. It will also provide some historical background to the problems encountered by sportspersons as counsel to those who have used or might anticipate using these drugs, albeit inadvertently.

## ASTHMA AND ITS TREATMENT

Asthma is a chronic inflammatory disorder of the airways. In susceptible individuals this inflammation causes recurrent episodes of coughing, wheezing, chest tightness and dyspnoea. Inflammation makes the airways sensitive to stimuli such as allergens, chemical irritants, tobacco smoke, cold air or exercise. When exposed to these stimuli, the airways may become swollen, constricted, filled with mucus and hyper-responsive to stimuli. The resulting airflow limitation is reversible (but not completely so in some patients), either spontaneously or with treatment. When asthma therapy is adequate, inflammation can be reduced over the long term, symptoms can usually be controlled and most asthma-related problems prevented.

### Epidemiology

Asthma is one of the commonest chronic conditions. It affects children more commonly than adults. It is estimated that 1 in 7 children (ages 2-15) and 1 in 25 adults (aged 16 and over) in the UK has asthma symptoms currently requiring treatment. That is equivalent to 1.5 million children and 1.9 million adults. The global incidence of asthma is estimated to be 100 million.

### Pathophysiology

An asthma attack always consists of an early phase and frequently contains a late phase. The early phase occurs within minutes of exposure to the trigger factor, reaches a maximum in 15-20 minutes and normally resolves within an hour. It is caused by bronchoconstriction. The late phase occurs 2-4 hours after exposure to the trigger factor and reaches a maximum after 6-8 hours. It is caused by inflammation of the airways.

Historically, it was thought that airway obstruction and hence difficulty of breathing in asthma were caused by contraction of airway smooth muscle, i.e. bronchoconstriction. However, post-mortem findings in asthma have revealed the cardinal features of inflammation.

There is disruption of the airway epithelium (desquamation) and exposure of subepithelial tissue. The subepithelium demonstrates increased blood flow (hyperaemia), oedema (caused by increased vascular permeability), hypertrophy of airway smooth muscle and accumulations of pro-inflammatory cells (particularly eosinophils and mononuclear cells). The molecular mechanisms of the inflammation are extremely complex and not fully understood. The putative mediators of asthma parallel the chronology of the discovery of inflammatory mediators.

Thus they have changed from histamine to the cyclo-oxygenase-mediated metabolites of arachidonic acid, to platelet-activating factor and currently to the lipoxygenase-mediated metabolites of arachidonic acid (namely the leukotrienes). It is unlikely that the inflammatory processes in asthma can be attributed to either a single mediator or a family of mediators. Nevertheless, appreciation of the change of emphasis from bronchoconstriction to inflammation as the cause of airway obstruction has underpinned the change in approach to the management of asthma as defined by organizations such as the British Thoracic Society.

## TRIGGER FACTORS

There are numerous factors which can trigger an asthma attack. The commonest are allergens. These can be either inhaled, such as pollens and/or animal danders (hairs and feathers), or ingested, such as dairy produce or strawberries. Viral, but not bacterial, infection of the upper respiratory tract can trigger asthma. Indeed, the initial presenting feature of asthma may be a persistent wheeze after a self-limiting, upper respiratory tract, viral infection. Occupational pollution can cause asthma. The National Asthma Campaign suggests that the true figure may be nearer 1500-2000 new cases per annum. Asthma attacks can be precipitated by emotional factors. This should not be misinterpreted as an indication that asthma is psychosomatic.

Rather it is a reflection of neuroendocrine changes which, as yet, are poorly understood. Certain drugs may precipitate an asthma attack. Beta blockers and non-steroidal anti-inflammatory drugs (NSAIDs), particularly aspirin, can evoke a potentially fatal asthmatic attack. Beta blockers cause bronchoconstriction by blocking the bronchodilating β2 -receptors on airway smooth muscle. They should not be administered to asthmatics. The mechanism by which NSAIDs evoke bronchospasm is hypothetical but may involve a shift in balance between bronchodilating and bronchoconstricting metabolites of arachidonic acid.

Approximately 10 per cent of asthmatics are aspirin sensitive and will develop bronchoconstriction if given the drug. For this reason, aspirin and other NSAIDs should be used with caution in asthmatics. Finally, and most importantly in the context of sport, exercise can cause bronchoconstriction, in which case exercise-induced asthma (EIA) is diagnosed. An asthmatic may be sensitive to a variety of trigger factors or to just one.

## MANAGEMENT OF ASTHMA

Non-drug treatment of asthma involves avoidance of known trigger factors. Drug treatment of asthma is now directed at arresting and reversing the inflammatory process. The emphasis has shifted from the excessive and inappropriate use of β2 -agonist bronchodilator therapy towards the early use of anti-inflammatory drugs. β2 -Agonists merely relieve the symptoms of asthma without addressing the underlying inflammation.

This has been likened to 'painting over rust'. Guidelines for treatment of chronic asthma have been prepared in several countries including Britain and the United States. They constitute a systematic approach to the treatment of increasing severity of symptoms. It must be remembered that the treatment of asthma can also be stepped down if the severity of the symptoms declines.

**Step 1**

Occasional use of relief bronchodilators Inhaled short-acting β2 -agonists should be used as required. If they are needed more than once daily or there are nocturnal symptoms.

**Step 2**

Regular inhaled anti-inflammatory drugs

Inhaled short-acting β2 -agonists as required plus

Either standard-dose inhaled corticosteroid (e.g. beclomethasone or budesonide (100-400 μg twice daily) or cromoglycate or nedocromil (mast cell stabilizers). If control of symptoms is not achieved then inhaled steroids should be substituted for the mast cell stabilizer. N.B. A higher dose of inhaled corticosteroid may be needed to gain initial control of symptoms. A doubling of the dose may be needed to gain control during acute exacerbations.

**Step 3**

High-dose inhaled corticosteroids or standard-dose inhaled corticosteroids and long-acting inhaled β2-agonists Inhaled short-acting β2 -agonists as required plusEither regular high-dose inhaled corticosteroid [beclomethasone or budesonide (up to a maximum of 800-2000 μg daily in divided doses) or fluticasone (up to 1000 μg daily in divided doses)] via a large volume spacer. Or regular standard-dose inhaled corticosteroid plus regular inhaled long-acting β2 -agonist (salmeterol 50 μg twice daily or in those over 18 years, formoterol 12 μg twice daily).

**Step 4**

High-dose inhaled steroids and regular bronchodilators Inhaled short-acting β2 -agonists as required Plus regular high-dose inhaled corticosteroid Plus sequential therapeutic trial of one or more of the following:

*Long-acting inhaled β2 -agonist*

*Modified-release oral theophylline*
*Inhaled ipratropium or, in adults, oxitropium*
*Modified-release oral β2 -agonists*
*High-dose inhaled β2 -agonist*
*Cromoglycate or nedocromil.*

**Step 5**

Regular corticosteroid tablets Inhaled short-acting β2 -agonists as required Plus regular high-dose inhaled corticosteroid And one or more of the long-acting bronchodilators Plus regular prednisolone tablets. N.B. In addition to regular prednisolone, continue high-dose inhaled corticosteroid.

**Stepping down**

Treatment should be reviewed every three to six months. If the patient has been stable during that period then it may be possible to introduce a slow, stepwise reduction in therapy. If treatment started recently at Step 4 or 5, then the reduction may take place after a short interval. In other patients, a 1-3-month period of stability is needed before stepwise reduction is undertaken.

## PHARMACOLOGY OF ANTI-ASTHMA DRUGS

## ANTI-INFLAMMATORY DRUGS

There are three groups of drugs which are used prophylactically, i.e. to prevent an asthma attack from occurring. They do not dilate a constricted airway and should not be used for symptomatic relief during an acute asthma attack. They are referred to colloquially as 'preventers'.

## SODIUM CROMOGLYCATE (SCG)

Administration is by inhalation of dry powder, by aerosol or nebulizer. SCG is better tolerated than inhaled corticosteroids but less effective. Side-effects are rare. Infrequently, a slight cough, bronchospasm or throat irritation can be caused by inhalation of the dry powder. This can be circumvented either by using an aerosol or more simply by drinking a little water after administration of the drug. Alternatively, a short-acting β2 -agonist can be inhaled shortly before SCG. SCG is effective in 40-50 per cent of children but relatively ineffective in adults.

The mode of action is controversial. The classical explanation is that SCG stabilizes the membrane of mast cells and prevents the release of the mediators of inflammation and bronchoconstriction. However, other mast cell stabilizers have been ineffective in the treatment of asthma. There is an increasing volume of evidence which suggests that the anti-inflammatory activity of SCG may be attributable to inhibition of airway sensory receptors and hence of neurogenic inflammation of the airways. It must be emphasized to the patient that SCG prevents airway inflammation but does not dilate constricted airways. Consequently, it will not relieve the symptoms of an attack.

Hence, SCG should be used regularly to prevent attacks and not to relieve symptoms of an established attack. If this is not explained to the patient then they may dismiss the drug as being ineffective. The duration of action is 2-4 hours. Nedocromil sodium, a derivative of SCG, has a similar profile of activity but a longer duration of action (6-12 hours). SCG has no effect on the cardiovascular system and is of no ergogenic value. It should be used from Step 2 onwards of the British Thoracic Society guidelines for the treatment of asthma. Its use is permitted by the IOC.

### Corticosteroids

Glucocorticosteroids (GCS) are the mainstay of the treatment of chronic asthma in both children and adults. They are also a quintessential component of the emergency treatment of acute severe asthma in both children and adults. At the molecular level they increase the synthesis of anti-inflammatory mediators. Therapeutically, they decrease the swelling and oedema of the inflamed bronchial mucosa, reduce mucus secretion and airway hypersensitivity, whilst increasing the sensitivity to β2 -agonists. Steroids may be administered by inhalation, orally, or by injection. Inhaled steroids are the anti-inflammatory drugs of choice for the prophylaxis of chronic asthma. It is estimated that 3 per cent of the total population in the UK is currently taking an inhaled steroid. Moreover, approximately one-fifth of these patients or 333000 are using doses in excess of 1000 μg a day.

The dose that is used should be the minimum that is commensurate with satisfactory control of symptoms. Because budesonide and fluticasone have a longer duration of action than beclomethasone, they need only be administered twice daily, whereas beclomethasone may be administered up to a maximum of 4 times daily. Together with β2 -agonists inhaled corticosteroids account for almost 90 per cent of UK prescriptions for asthma. The glucocorticoid group of steroid hormones do not have an anabolic effect. Inhaled/ topical steroids do not have a positive ergogenic effect and are permitted by the IOC. Systemic administration of glucocorticosteroids, i.e. orally (e.g. prednisolone), rectally or by either intravenous or intramuscular injection (e.g. hydrocortisone), is prohibited by the IOC.

## Leukotriene Antagonists

Leukotrienes (LTs) are a family of lipid mediators derived from arachidonic acid by the action, initially, of the enzyme 5-lipoxygenase. LTs are released from pro-inflammatory cells in response to a variety of stimuli and can evoke many of the cardinal features of asthma, such as increased mucus production, airway wall oedema, eosinophil accumulation and activation, and bronchoconstriction. Leukotriene antagonists selectively block the receptors for a sub-group of LTs, the cysteinyl leukotrienes.

There are currently two drugs licensed in the UK, montelukast and zafirlukast. When they were licensed in 1998 they were the first novel treatment for asthma in 25 years. They are orally active, which is an advantage over existing inhaled medications because it is more convenient and may help patient compliance with therapy. However, they should be considered as add-on therapy for those patients with mild to moderate asthma that is not controlled with an inhaled corticosteroid and a short-acting β2 -agonist. In the UK, the Committee on Safety of Medicines (CSM) has advised that LT antagonists should not be used to relieve an attack of acute severe asthma and that their use does not necessarily allow a reduction in existing corticosteroid treatment. Their use is permitted by the IOC.

## Bronchodilator Drugs

There are three groups of drugs which are used to relax the constricted airways of the asthmatic during an attack. These drugs are used to treat the symptoms of asthma, rather than to prevent an attack from occurring. They are referred to colloquially as 'relievers'.

### SELECTIVE B2-ADRENOCEPTOR AGONISTS

The first β-agonist to be used in the treatment of asthma was isoprenaline. The increase in asthma mortality which paralleled the introduction of isoprenaline prompted the development of a new generation of selective β2 -agonists for use as bronchodilators. There are currently six selective β2-agonists licensed in the UK for the treatment of asthma.

All the selective β2 -agonists are potent bronchodilators. They differ in their time to onset and duration of action. Salbutamol and terbutaline are short acting and the most frequently used β2 -agonists in the UK. There are many formulations of salbutamol and terbutaline including tablets, slow-release tablets, elixirs, aerosols and dry powder, solutions for injection and inhalation from a nebulizer. Inhalation is the route of choice because it is the most rapidly effective (1-2 minutes) and is associated with the fewest side-effects.

Tremor is the only common side-effect after inhalation. The side-effects after oral administration include: fine tremor nervous tension and headache. Tachycardia, peripheral vasodilation and hypokalaemia may occur after oral dosing but are commoner after intravenous injection. Tachycardia is most common after nebulization. The duration of action of salbutamol and terbutaline after aerosol administration is approximately 4 hours. Formoterol (eformoterol) and salmeterol are the most frequently prescribed long-acting β2 -agonists with a duration of action of approximately 12 hours.

The properties of different β2 -agonists determine their use in the treatment of asthma. Rapid-onset, short-acting β2 -agonists areused to give immediate and/or emergency relief from symptoms. There are differences between the time to onset of action for formoterol and salmeterol. The former begins to take effect within 1-3 minutes whilst the latter takes 10-20 minutes. Nevertheless, long-acting β2 -agonists should not be used for immediate relief of symptoms.

***Table:*** Selective β2-adrenoceptor agonists

| |
|---|
| Salbutamol (Ventolin™) |
| Terbutaline (Bricanyl™) |
| Bambuterol (Bambec™) |
| Fenoterol (Berotec™) |
| Formoterol/Eformoterol (Foradil™/Oxis™) |
| Salmeterol (Serevent™) |

Instead, they should be used in addition to inhaled corticosteroids to treat troublesome nocturnal symptoms and to prevent exercise-induced asthma when their longer duration of action confers a definite advantage. What is more, their respective role in the management of asthma is still evolving. It was thought that short-acting b2 -agonists should be used to a maximum of 4 times a day. However, this provides no clear clinical benefit when compared with their use 'as required'. Indeed, a recent clinical trial has shown greater efficacy of formoterol compared with terbutaline when used 'as required' in terms of improved lung function, symptoms and quality of life. This has considerable cost implications since long-acting b2 -agonists are considerably more expensive than short-acting b2 -agonists.

The use of β2 -agonists is governed by IOC Regulations. Historically, controversy over the use of sympathomimetics has centred upon the potential ergogenic value of the cardiovascular and central nervous system side-effects that these drugs can evoke. Thus, α-agonists, non-selective α/β-agonists and non-selective β-agonists are included in Class 1A (stimulants) of the IOC Prohibited Classes of Substances. The 1992 Olympics in Barcelona turned the spotlight on to a new controversy surrounding selective β2 -agonists, namely the putative anabolic effects of β2 -agonists, in general, and clenbuterol in particular. Two British weightlifters were withdrawn from the Olympic Games that year when they tested positive for clenbuterol.

A USA competitor and a German athlete also tested positive and were banned for using clenbuterol. In July 1992, the IOC classification of selective β2 -agonists was changed radically. Only salbutamol and terbutaline were permitted and then only by inhalation and following written notification to the relevant medical authority by the team physician. All β2 -agonists, except salbutamol and terbutaline, were re-classified into sub-group 2 (other anabolic agents) of Doping Class C Anabolic Agents. This sub-group included only β2 -agonists and specified clenbuterol as the example. Since 1992 there have been several positive tests for clenbuterol. In 1997, Djamolidin Abduzhaparov tested positive in the Tour de France and was withdrawn. Clenbuterol was one of the frequently used drugs cited by Willy Voet in his account of the notorious Festina Affair' in the 1998 Tour de France. In 1999, two Chinese swimmers received 3-year bans after testing positive for the second time. In the 2000 Olympic games in Sydney, there was one positive test upon which no action was taken because there had been prior notification of use.

Clenbuterol is a long-acting β2 -agonist which is licensed for the treatment of asthma in several countries including Germany, Italy and Spain. The drug is available in a variety of formulations including syrup, aerosol, injectable solutions and granules. It is not licensed for human use in either the UK or the USA. It is licensed for veterinary use in horses for the treatment of bronchoconstriction caused by several equine respiratory diseases. The therapeutic dose for the treatment of asthma is 20-30 μg per day. It is misused in humans as an anabolic agent when doses of 100-140 μg per day are commonly employed. It is widely available on the Internet and the 'black market'. The maximum effective dose is limited by availability of β2 -receptors. One of the advantages of clenbuterol is that it is not a steroid and therefore does not cause steroid-related side-effects. However, it is a β2 -agonist and has side-effects which are typical of this group of drugs, i.e. tremor, restlessness, agitation, headache, increased blood pressure and palpitations. These side-effects are dose-related and purported to decrease after 8-10 days.

This is due to a decrease, i.e. down-regulation, of β2 -receptors, a consequence of which is also a decrease in the anabolic effect of the drug. This has resulted in various dose-cycle regimens being adopted by abusers, details of which are readily available on the Internet. The 'off periods are often associated with withdrawal symptoms as the CNS stimulant effects decline. There is anecdotal evidence that a variety of sympathomimetic drugs have been used to attenuate the severity of the withdrawal symptoms.

Colloquially, clenbuterol is described as either a 'fat burner' or a 'repartitioning agent'. In the high doses at which the drug is abused, it is reported to increase non-shivering thermogenesis by increasing metabolism in brown fat. A 1° increase of body temperature will increase basal calorific utilization by 5 per cent. Because of the effect upon metabolic rate, clenbuterol is contraindicated in people with hyperthyroidism. In addition β3 -agonists activate lipolysis in fat cells. The evidence for the anabolic effect of clenbuterol in animals is considerable. It increases muscle mass by causing hypertrophy but not hyperplasia. It inhibits muscle protein catabolism, which is why it is reported to be abused in humans after discontinuation of steroids to reduce the catabolic phase. The combination of an increase in lipolysis and an increase in muscle mass results in an increase in lean body mass, hence the description of 'a repartitioning agent'.

The current regulations regarding the use of β2 -agonists are explained in the Olympic Movement Anti-Doping Code (OMAC). The only β2 -agonists that are permitted within Class 1A Stimulants are formoterol, salbutamol, salmeterol and terbutaline. The use of these drugs is restricted to inhaler only to prevent and/or treat asthma and exercise-induced asthma. Written notification to the relevant medical authority, by a respiratory or team physician, of asthma and/or exercise-induced asthma is necessary prior to competition. At the

Olympic Games in Salt Lake City, athletes who required an inhaled β2 -agonist to treat asthma and/or exercise-induced bronchoconstriction (exercise-induced 'asthma') were required to submit to the IOC-MC clinical and laboratory (including respiratory function tests) evidence that justified such treatment. This had to be received by the IOC-MC at least 1 week prior to the athlete's first competition.

A panel of scientific and medical experts reviewed the submitted information. In doubtful cases, the panel had the authority to perform appropriate scientifically validated tests. All other β2 -agonists are prohibited under Class C Anabolic Agents: 2. β2 –Agonists. The definition of a positive test for salbutamol as a stimulant is a urine concentration greater than 100 nanograms/ml and as an anabolic agent, 1000 ng/ml.

## METHYL XANTHINES

Both theophylline and aminophylline (the soluble ethylenediamine-derivative of theophylline) are related to caffeine. They are classed as additional bronchodilators and should be confined to Stages 3,4 and 5 of the BTS Guidelines. They constitute the second line of bronchodilator therapy. They must be given orally or intravenously and the risk of side-effects is much greater than with selective β2 -agonists. The dose should be adjusted to provide a therapeutic plasma theophylline concentration of 10-20 μg/ml.

Although the absolute threshold varies between individuals, both the frequency and severity of side-effects increases with the plasma concentration. Thus 15 μg/ ml is associated with nausea, vomiting, abdominal pains, headache, nervousness and muscle tremor. Plasma concentrations between 20 and 40 μg/ml can cause convulsions and ventricular arrhythmias increasing in severity from tachycardia to fibrillation and ultimately cardiac arrest. Sustained-release tablets are now the formulation of choice because they have reduced the fluctuations in plasma concentrations of theophylline and hence have reduced the incidence of side-effects. Cardiovascular side-effects are associated more with theophylline and central nervous system side-effects with caffeine. Caffeine is banned by the IOC if the urinary concentration exceeds 12 μg/ml.

Their mode of action is contentious. The classical explanation is that they inhibit phosphodiesterase, the enzyme responsible for the inactivation of cAMP. However, the plasma concentration required to achieve this inhibition in vivo is a factor of 10 times the accepted upper limit of therapeutic plasma concentrations. Alternatively, there is evidence that methyl xanthines antagonize adenosine receptors. Theophylline and aminophylline also down-regulate the activity of pro-inflammatory cells. Whatever the mode of action, these drugs have a place in treatment of both chronic and acute severe asthma. The methyl xanthines are permitted by the IOC.

## Anticholinergic Drugs

The parasympathetic nervous system causes contraction of bronchial smooth muscle by the effect of acetylcholine upon muscarinic cholinergic receptors. Theoretically, therefore, anticholinergic drugs should be of benefit in the treatment of asthma. In practice, they have a greater bronchodilator effect in chronic bronchitics than in asthmatics. Inhaled ipratropium bromide, which is a quaternary derivative of atropine, is a useful alternative for individuals who cannot tolerate or respond to β2-agoinsts- It is classed as an additional bronchodilator and should be used in Stage 4 or 5 of the BTS Guidelines. It has a slow onset time (30-60 min) and is active for 3-4 hours and hence should be taken four times per day. Oxitropium bromide, a derivative of ipratropium, has a longer duration of action and need only be taken twice daily. Neither drug will give rapid relief of symptoms.

The side-effects of antagonism of the parasympathetic nervous system are dry mouth, urinary retention and constipation. However, ipratropium bromide is poorly absorbed and is not associated with significant side-effects when standard doses are administered by inhalation. The IOC permits the use of ipratropium bromide for the treatment of asthma.

## EXERCISE AND ASTHMA

Asthma presents a twofold problem to elite sportspersons. First, it can impair performance if not treated correctly. However, many athletes compete successfully at the highest level despite asthma, for example Paula Radcliffe who captained the British female athletes at the Sydney Olympics and who is the 2002 Commonwealth 5000 m, European 10 000 m and long-course, World cross-country champion. Second and perhaps of greater concern, treatment can expose the sportsperson to drugs which are contained in the OMAC lists of Prohibited Classes of Substances.

The incidence of asthma is reported to be more common in elite athletes than in the general population. In 1984, it was reported that 11.2 per cent of US athletes competing in the Los Angeles Olympics had exercise-induced asthma. A second study was undertaken of 699 athletes prior to the 1996 Summer Olympics in Atlanta: 16.7 per cent had a history of asthma, took anti-asthma medications or both; 10.4 per cent had active asthma. This compares with 3-7 per cent of the general population in the USA.

Exercise may be one of a number of trigger factors for an individual's asthma or it may be the only trigger factor. This led to the concept of exercise-induced asthma (EIA) as a syndrome discrete from asthma. Thus, EIA has been defined in terms of the trigger factor, i.e. as reversible airway obstruction that occurs during or after exertion. The initial response to exercise in both non-asthmatics and asthmatics is bronchodilation.

However, in the asthmatic, initial bronchodilation is not sustained and bronchoconstriction develops, most dramatically once the exercise has been terminated. The maximum decrease in peak expiratory flow rate (PEFR) and forced expiratory volume in the first second (FEV1) normally occur between 3 and 15 minutes after the exercise has been completed. The ventilatory changes in EIA are identical to those observed during a spontaneous asthma attack, i.e. decreased Vt (tidal volume), PEFR, FEV1, FVC (forced vital capacity) and increased residual volume (RV) leading to hyperventilation and dyspnoea.

The symptoms include coughing, wheezing, excessive sputum production, dyspnoea and/or chest tightness. All of these changes are observed in asthma induced by factors other than exercise. In the laboratory, the exercise needs to be of 6-8 minutes duration at greater than 80 per cent of predicted maximal heart rate although in their sport, the early phase may take longer to develop. The maximum decrease in lung function occurs after 15 minutes and returns towards normal function after approximately one hour. This is known as the early phase of EIA. EIA may consist of just an early phase or, in approximately 30 per cent of EIA patients, may also develop a late phase after 6-8 hours.

In 50 per cent of individuals affected by EIA, a second period of exercise within 2 hours of the initial period evokes a weaker bronchoconstrictor response. The period during which the response is less is referred to as the refractory period. Advantage can be taken of the refractory period for both training and competition. Exercise-induced asthma occurs in up to 90 per cent of people with chronic asthma and 40 per cent of people with allergic rhinitis. A 23 per cent incidence of exercise-induced asthma was found among 1998 US Winter Olympians. Random testing of asymptomatic children found that 7 per cent had EIA.

The pathophysiology of EIA is only partially understood. It is accepted that the severity of EIA is dependent upon the level of ventilation and the temperature and humidity of the inspired air. Cold dry air is more asthmogenic than warm humid air. This challenges the homeostatic regulation of airway temperature and water loss. Water loss from the airway epithelial cells decreases the cell volume and increases the viscosity of mucus. The latter can obstruct airflow and stimulate the cough reflex. After the challenge has subsided, the airways must be re-warmed and the intracellular fluid that was lost must be replaced. This can cause reactive hyperaemia (increased blood flow to the airway wall) and rebound increase in cell volume. This may be the key event that causes release of mediators and triggers bronchoconstriction and inflammatory changes in the airway wall. It may also explain the time course of the changes in lung function. Moreover, cycling may be the most asthmogenic sport because both training and competition involve longer periods of challenge to the respiratory tract.

Typical cycling road races can last in excess of 4 hours whereas marathons last 2.5 hours and football matches last 1.5 hours. Finally, the environment in which the exercise takes place is important. Thus cross-country skiing, which is conducted in cold dry air environments, has one of the highest incidences of reported EIA.

### Treatment of Exercise-induced Asthma (EIA)

The management of EIA consists of both non-drug and drug interventions and is directed at two goals: optimal control of base-line symptoms and prevention of an asthmatic attack following exercise. Relief of symptoms of EIA should be considered as an indication that the first two goals have not been achieved satisfactorily.

## NON-DRUG TREATMENT

### Aerobic Fitness

Fitness does not prevent EIA as indicated by the number of Olympians who suffer from the syndrome. However, aerobic fitness does improve lung function, retards deterioration in lung function with age (in non-asthmatics) and enables asthmatics to exercise with less EIA. It also facilitates social interactions and improves self-esteem of asthmatics. There is no evidence to suggest that aerobic training is deleterious to asthmatics provided that their treatment is optimal and that they have a satisfactory management plan which includes access to appropriate bronchodilator therapy, if required. The only contraindication for strenuous aerobic activity in an asthmatic would be if they demonstrated significant arterial desaturation upon exercise-testing during laboratory investigations.

## Minimize Cooling and Drying of the Airways

This can be achieved in several ways. First, if possible, select a physical activity such as walking and swimming which are less likely to evoke bronchoconstriction. Second, utilize nasal breathing whenever possible. Third, seek to avoid exercising in a cold, dry environment. If this is unavoidable then a face mask may reduce cooling and drying of the airways.

## Warm-up

This can help to maximize the benefit of the training session and, if possible, should take cognizance of the refractory period that many asthmatics experience after an initial episode of EIA. The warm-up should be of 15 minutes' duration. It is debatable whether this should involve high intensity bursts to increase ventilation rapidly or moderate sustained activity. It is also advisable to cool down gradually after the exercise to minimize rebound warming of the airways.

## Monitoring of PEFR

This will provide objective assessment of the current status of base-line control of asthma. Inadequate base-line control requires revision of maintenance therapy. Concurrent conditions such as hay fever and allergic rhinitis should also be satisfactorily controlled. If possible, training and participation should not be undertaken on days when symptoms are poorly controlled.

## Drug Treatment

The treatment of EIA focuses upon prevention rather than relief of symptoms. β2 -Agonists and mast cell stabilizers are the most effective and proven therapies for the prevention of EIA.

## β2-Agonists

These drugs are the most effective prophylactic treatment of EIA. Salbutamol, terbutaline and salmeterol are the only β2 -agonists which are permitted by the IOC. Short-acting β2 -agonists (i.e. salbutamol or terbutaline) should be administered 15 to 30 minutes before commencing exercise. They induce bronchodilation within 5 minutes and afford protection against EIA for approximately 3-6 hours. They prevent asthma symptoms in 90 per cent of patients. They should be available to the athlete for rapid relief of symptoms should they develop despite pre-exercise treatment. Salmeterol, a long-acting β2 -agonist, should be taken 30 minutes before exercise and is effective for up to 9 hours.

It is licensed in the UK for the treatment of troublesome nocturnal symptoms and exercise-induced asthma. Its long duration of action makes it suitable for children who require prophylaxis against EIA throughout the school day. Because of its slower onset of action, salmeterol should not be used as a rescue medication to relieve symptoms of an asthma attack. Salbutamol or terbutaline should be used instead. There is controversy about the relative merits of the long-term prophylactic use of short- and long-acting β2 -agonists. Tachyphylaxis to salmeterol has been shown to develop after 4 weeks of regular use. Alternatives to regular use of salmeterol are either short-acting β2 -agonists before exercise and 'on-demand' for relief of symptoms or leukotriene antagonists before exercise.

## MAST CELL STOBILIZERS

Sodium cromoglycate (SCG) and nedocromil sodium are the next most effective and most frequently used drugs for the treatment of EIA. It should be remembered that neither SCG nor nedocromil sodium is a bronchodilator. They are anti-inflammatories and are used prophylactically to prevent EIA. Neither drug is as effective as short-acting β2 -agonists which also prevent EIA, but by causing bronchodilation.

They should be administered 10-15 minutes before the start of exercise and will provide up to two hours' protection against bronchoconstriction. They prevent asthma symptoms in 70-85 per cent of patients with EIA. SCG is often extremely effective when combined with a short-acting β2 -agonist in those patients for whom monotherapy is ineffective. Neither SCG nor nedocromil sodium is included in the lists of Prohibited Substances and Prohibited Methods. It should be noted that sodium cromoglycate is available as a compound formulation with salbutamol. This preparation is not recommended because it may be used inappropriately to relieve symptoms, whereas it should be used prophylactically.

## METHYL XANTHINES

Theophylline is administered orally either as a rapid-release or a sustained-release formulation. The rapid-release formulation must be administered 1-2 hours before exercise. The narrow therapeutic window of theophylline coupled with the many factors that can affect plasma concentrations and either increase toxicity or decrease efficacy of the drug mean that it is impracticable to administer a single dose as a prophylactic against EIA.

The sustained-release formulation is used prophylactically in order to maintain better base-line control of asthma in accordance with BTS Guidelines. The aforementioned factors, together with the greater risk of cardiovascular and CNS side-effects from theophylline, compared with either inhaled short-acting β2 -agonists or mast cell stabilizers, relegates theophylline to the third line of therapy for EIA. Theophylline is not included in the OMAC lists of Prohibited Substances and Prohibited Methods.

### Corticosteroids

The time to onset of anti-inflammatory effects of inhaled steroids is 8-12 hours. Hence, single doses of inhaled steroids immediately prior to exercise do not afford protection against EIA. A 4-week trial of inhaled betamethasone valerate produced a significant improvement in EIA, but this was probably related to better base-line control of asthma. Inhaled budesonide twice a day for 4 weeks produced a significant improvement in resting pulmonary function and in the benefit derived from pre-exercise terbutaline. The role of inhaled steroids in the treatment of EIA is now considered to be in the establishment of satisfactory base-line control of symptoms.

## ANTICHOLINERGICS

These drugs are of minor importance in the treatment of EIA. Broncho-dilatation produced by inhalation of 0.5 mg of ipratropium bromide was equal to that of a β2 -agonist, but was not effective against EIA. Two studies have demonstrated a synergistic effect between SCG and ipratropium bromide in the treatment of EIA. However, ipratropium bromide alone does not compare with β2 -agonists in either the prevention or the reversal of EIA. Neither ipratropium nor its longer-acting derivative, oxitropium, is included in the OMAC lists of Prohibited Substances and Prohibited Methods.

### Leukotriene antagonists

In the UK, montelukast and zafirlukast are licensed for the prophylaxis of asthma. In the USA, an inhibitor of LT synthesis, zileuton, is also marketed. For this reason, in the USA, the group of drugs is referred to as LT modifiers rather than simply as the LT antagonists. It is suggested that LT antagonists may be of benefit in preventing exercise-induced asthma and in those asthmatics who are aspirin sensitive. An 8-week, multicentre, randomized, double-blind comparison of oral, once daily, montelukast (10 mg) with inhaled, twice daily (50 μg) salmeterol showed that montelukast provided consistent long-term protection against EIA without tachyphylaxis. A significant loss of protection was seen over the 8-week period with salmeterol.

Montelukast offers several advantages over other prophylactic therapies. First, it is available as a once daily, oral medication. In those who respond, it is effective for up to 20-24 hours. It is permitted by the IOC without prior notification. However, there are two potential disadvantages. First, not all patients will respond and the figure may be as high as 75 per cent. Second, Churg-Strauss syndrome has been reported, albeit rarely, in association with the use of LT antagonists. Whilst a causal relationship may not have been established and the possibility exists that the syndrome may be caused by reduction or withdrawal of corticosteroids, the CSM advises that patients be informed and alerted to the possible risks.

## TREATMENT OF COUGHS AND COLDS

Cough is a protective reflex that is initiated by either mechanical or chemical stimulation of the oral pharynx, larynx, trachea or bronchi. Its purpose is to remove mucus and irritants from the upper respiratory tract (URT). Most commonly it is a symptom of a self-limiting URT infection that will normally resolve, without treatment, within 3-4 days. Antibiotics are of no value because the infection is normally viral and not bacterial. There is evidence to support a causal link between intense exercise and the incidence of URT infection. In the case of male endurance runners, there appears to be a dose-related effect of exercise training on the risk of URT infection.

This relationship is highlighted by the T curve model proposed by Nieman whereby the risk of URT infection is reduced below that of sedentary individuals when engaged in mild to moderate intensity exercise training and increased when engaged in high intensity exercise training. However, a direct link between infection and disturbed immune function in athletes has not been fully established.

Less frequently, cough is a symptom of serious disease of the respiratory tract (e.g. chronic obstructive pulmonary disease, tuberculosis and bronchial carcinoma), but this is unlikely to be relevant to an individual who is participating in top level competitive sport. However, this was most certainly not the case with Lance Armstrong, four times winner of the Tour de France, whose cough was a symptom of pulmonary metastases secondary to testicular cancer.

The important therapeutic distinction is between productive and non-productive coughs. A productive cough should not be suppressed but should be facilitated by adequate fluid intake and, possibly, with the use of an expectorant. A non-productive cough may be suppressed or perhaps converted into a productive cough by increased fluid intake and the use of either an expectorant or, in exceptional circumstances, a mucolytic.

The number of OTC (over-the-counter or non-prescription) medications available for the treatment of coughs and colds is enormous. The global market for 1999 was valued at $6.5 bn. There are approximately 500 OTC cough and cold preparations available in the USA. There are approximately 160 OTC cough and cold preparations in the UK with a market value of £337.4 million in 1999. The majority of these preparations contain more than one active ingredient, some of which are banned by the IOC, for example sympathomimetics and narcotic analgesics.

Therefore, great care must be taken by the sportsperson when purchasing a cough or cold remedy for consumption at a time when they may be subject to testing under IOC or related regulations. The major classes of drugs which are contained in cough and cold preparations are: cough suppressants, sympathomimetics, expectorants, demulcents, and xanthines.

## Cough Suppressants

There are two groups of centrally active cough suppressants: narcotic analgesics and antihistamines. Centrally acting cough suppressants reduce coughing by inhibiting the cough centre in the medulla oblongata in the brainstem. The three main drugs in this category are the opioid derivatives, codeine, pholcodine and dextromethorphan.

They can each cause drowsiness, respiratory depression and constipation. Codeine is a narcotic analgesic which can cause both physical and psychological dependence and hence potentially is a drug of abuse. However, the antitussive dose (normally 15-30 mg, 3-4 times a day) is less than that required for analgesia and the risk of unwitting addiction is merely theoretical.

Pholcodine has less potential for addiction and causes less respiratory depression and constipation than codeine. For these reasons, it is preferable to codeine as a cough suppressant. The recommended daily dose is 5-10 mg, 3-4 times a day. Dextromethorphan was introduced in 1958 and is essentially free of analgesic and addictive properties and causes less respiratory depression and constipation than either codeine or pholcodine. It is available in many OTC cough and cold preparations and is the safest of the three cough suppressants. The recommended daily dose is 10-30 mg, 3-4 times a day. The use of all three centrally acting cough suppressants (codeine, pholcodine and dextromethorphan) is permitted by the IOC.

However, although these drugs are widely available for cough suppression and are permitted by the IOC, there is scant justification for their use by a sportsperson. First, there is little conclusive evidence that they completely suppress a cough. Second, they can cause drowsiness and constipation. Third, it should be remembered that they should only be used to suppress a non-productive cough when a demulcent may be more appropriate and have fewer adverse side-effects.

Antihistamines are of potential value in the treatment of nasal allergies, particularly hay fever, and may reduce rhinorrhoea and sneezing. They are less effective than sympathomimetics in reducing nasal congestion associated with the common cold. They are present in many cough and cold remedies. Antihistamines reduce coughing by two mechanisms. First, they have a central suppressant action that is non-narcotic but which does suppress the cough reflex. Second, their anticholinergic action reduces the rate of mucus secretion. This can increase the viscosity of mucus, which is why antihistamines should be used with caution in asthmatics. The overall decrease in mucus production complements the effects of sympathomimetics, which is why the two groups of drugs are commonly combined in cough and cold preparations.

The older antihistamines, such as brompheniramine and chlorpheniramine, have greater sedative activity than the newer antihistamines, such as acrivastine and cetirizine. However, the former are most commonly contained in OTC cough and cold preparations whilst the latter are only contained in POMs (prescription-only medicines) for the treatment of hay fever and other allergies. The use of antihistamines is permitted by the IOC.

## Sympathomimetic amines

Drugs which mimic the effects of the endogenous mediators of the sympathetic nervous system (i.e. adrenaline and noradrenaline) are referred to as sympathomimetic amines. Sympathomimetic amines work through the stimulation of adrenoceptors. The response of any cell or organ to sympathomimetic amines is directly related to the density and proportion of α- and β-adrenoceptors present.

According to Hoffman and Lefkowitz the actions of sympathomimetic amines can be classified into the following types:

- Peripheral excitatory action on vascular smooth muscle in blood vessels supplying the skin, kidneys and mucous membranes and glandular smooth muscle in salivary and sweat glands;
- Peripheral inhibitory action on the smooth muscle of the gut wall, the bronchioles and the blood vessels supplying the skeletal muscles;
- Cardiac excitatory action, inducing increased heart rate and force of contraction;
- Metabolic actions, including increased rate of glycogenolysis in the liver and muscles and mobilization of free fatty acids from adipose tissue;
- Endocrine actions, including regulation of the secretion of insulin, renin and pituitary hormones;
- CNS actions, including respiratory stimulation, increased wakefulness, psychomotor activity and reduction in appetite; and
- Presynaptic actions resulting in the inhibition or facilitation of release of neurotransmitters such as acetylcholine and noradrenaline. Not all sympathomimetic amines display all of the actions mentioned to the same degree, and many of the differences in their effects are only quantitative.

The profile of effects of each sympathomimetic amine is determined by its relative affinity for the sub-groups of adrenoceptors and forms the basis for their classification.

β2 -Receptors are located on airway smooth muscle and cause bronchodilation when stimulated. α1 -Receptors are located on arterial smooth muscle and cause vasoconstriction when stimulated. Consequently, β2 -agonists (e.g. salbutamol) are used as bronchodilators to treat asthma whilst α1 -agonists (e.g. ephedrine) are used as vasoconstrictors to treat coughs and colds. The primary role of sympathomimetic amines in the treatment of coughs and colds is to act as a decongestant. When the mucous membrane lining the nose is irritated by infection (e.g. in the common cold) or allergy (e.g. in seasonal allergic rhinitis), the blood vessels supplying the membrane become enlarged.

**Table.** Sympathomimetic amines categorized according to the principal adrenoceptors that they stimulate

| Sympathomimetic amine | Principal adrenoceptor stimulated |
|---|---|
| Salbutamol | $\beta^2$ |
| Terbutaline | β2 |
| Clenbuterol | β2 |
| Ephedrine | α1 |
| Phenylephrine | α1 |
| Phenylpropanolamine | α1 |
| Pseudoephedrine | α1 |

This leads to fluid accumulation in the surrounding tissue and encourages the production of larger than normal amounts of mucus. As well as affecting the nasal passages, congestion can also occur in the sinuses resulting in sinusitis. α1 -Agonists cause constriction of the blood vessels, so reducing the swelling in the lining of the nose and sinuses and acting as decongestants.

The most widely available α1-agonists present in OTC medications are referred to collectively as the ephedrines. Ephedrines can be defined as those compounds that are either isomers or stereoisomers of ephedrine and include pseudoephedrine, norephedrine (phenylpropanolamine) and norpseudoephedrine (cathine). Phenylephrine, also a sympathomimetic, is also commonly found in OTC formulations. The ephedrines and phenylephrine pose several potential problems for the sportsperson. First, they can cause significant side-effects. Second, their use is prohibited by the IOC under Class 1A, Stimulants.

Third, they are of doubtful ergogenic value. Finally, the choice is enormous and even the names of the proprietary preparations can be misleading. There are many opportunities to make a costly mistake.

## POTENTIAL SIDE-EFFECTS OF SYMPATHOMIMETIC AMINES

The decongestants, although widely available in OTC preparations, are potent vasoconstrictors as evinced by their licensed indications. In the UK, ephedrine is licensed for the treatment of hypotension caused by spinal or epidural anaesthesia.

It should be used with caution in hypertensive patients. Phenylephrine is licensed for the treatment of acute hypertension and is contraindicated in hypertensive patients. Pseudoephedrine is available in OTC cough and cold preparations and in tablet form as a systemic decongestant. It has few sympathomimetic side-effects. Phenylpropanolamine (PPA), on the other hand, is the most controversial of the sympathomimetics available in OTC cough and cold preparations.

Its use has been linked with hypertensive reactions, cerebral haemorrhage and psychosis. It does not have a licensed indication within the BNF but is widely available in OTC cough and cold preparations. In the USA, it is also marketed as an appetite suppressor. A recent study has demonstrated an odds ratio for association between haemorrhagic stroke and the use of PPA of 1.23 for cough and cold preparations and 15.92 for appetite suppressants. This has led to the United States Food and Drugs Administration (FDA) taking steps to remove PPA from all drug products. It is considered that

***Table:*** Recommended maximal therapeutic doses of the four commonest decongestants in OTC decongestant preparations

| *Sympathomimetic* | *Single dose (mg/4 hours)* | *Daily dose (mg)* |
|---|---|---|
| Ephedrine | 25 | 100 |
| Phenylephrine | 10 | 40 |
| Phenylpropanolamine | 25 | 100 |
| Pseudoephedrine | 60 | 240 |

although the risk is small, it cannot be justified for treatment of minor ailments. The Committee on Safety of Medicines in the UK has not recommended a ban on PPA for two reasons. First, the drug is not marketed in appetite suppressants in the UK. Second, the maximum approved daily OTC dose in the UK is 100 mg compared with 150 mg in the USA.

It is obvious, therefore, from clinical data that, when taken orally, α1 -agonist sympathomimetic amines can evoke profound systemic cardiovascular side-effects. Moreover, these effects are both drug-specific and dose-dependent. The current recommended oral doses for the four commonest decongestants.

There have been numerous reports of the effects upon cardiovascular parameters of those sympathomimetic amines which are contained in OTC medicines. Thomas et al reported significant increases in heart rate and both systolic and diastolic blood pressure following administration of two proprietary cold cure preparations containing the equivalent of double the therapeutic dose of phenylpropanolamine. Increases in diastolic blood pressure to 100 mmHg or more were reported in 12 out of 37 subjects taking preparations containing 85 mg of phenylpropanolamine. However, only 4 out of 34 subjects reached 100 mmHg diastolic blood pressure following treatment with a lower dose of 50 mg of phenylpropanolamine.

Doses equivalent to over three to four times the recommended therapeutic dose of pseudoephedrine raised diastolic pressure above 90 mmHg. These results were in accord with two other studies. Bye et al reported significant increases in heart rate and systolic blood pressure following relatively high doses (180 and 120 mg) of pseudoephedrine. Empey et al found doses of 120 and 180 mg produced statistically significant increases in both pulse and systolic blood pressure. However, the increases were deemed to be clinically unimportant as they were quantitatively considerably less than might be expected to occur with either emotion or mild exercise.

Whilst several studies have reported increased cardiovascular stimulation following ingestion of ephedrines, it is evident that doses used were at least twice the recommended single therapeutic dose. The reports of the effects of ingestion of ephedrines in single therapeutic doses have been conflicting.

Thus Bye et al. found that a single dose of ephedrine (25 mg) significantly elevated both heart rate and systolic blood pressure. In the same study, a single dose of pseudoephedrine (60 mg) significantly elevated only systolic arterial blood pressure. Bright et al found only a non-significant rise in resting heart rate following a single therapeutic dose of pseudoephedrine. Empey et al. reported that ingestion of pseudoephedrine in a therapeutic dose of 60 mg provided maximal nasal decongestion without any cardiovascular or other side-effects.

Few researchers have examined the effects of multiple dosing regimes on cardiovascular parameters. Chester found significant increases in blood pressure following multiple, therapeutic dosing regimen for pseudoephedrine (i.e. six 60 mg doses over a 36-hour period) and phenylpropanolamine (i.e. six 25 mg doses over a 36-hour period). Bye et al. reported significant increases in heart rate but not systolic arterial blood pressure after three different dose regimes, one involving two different sustained-release formulations.

Prolonged administration of a sustained-release formulation of pseudoephedrine (180 mg twice daily for 2 weeks) increased heart rate and decreased systolic arterial blood pressure. The authors could only speculate at the possible explanations for these results and the variance from those in the earlier study. Other studies that have addressed prolonged usage of ephedrines have been conflicting. Goodman et al. found no significant increase in blood pressure following daily administration of a 75-mg controlled release preparation of phenylpropanolamine for a period of 7 days. In an extensive study by Noble, more than 400 obese patients were administered 50 mg of phenylpropanolamine three times a daily over a 12-week period. Results showed no significant increase in blood pressure when compared with placebo.

The bronchodilator effects of ephedrines have been less well documented than the cardiovascular effects as might be expected from their receptor affinities. Ephedrines exert their effect principally on the $\alpha 1$ -receptors on vascular smooth muscle with minimal effect on $\beta 2$ -receptors in the bronchial smooth muscle. There have been no published reports on the stimulatory effects of phenylpropanolamine; however, some brochodilation has been claimed following administration of supratherapeutic doses of ephedrine (60 mg) and pseudoephedrine (210 mg).

In terms of action on the CNS, most evidence suggests that ephedrines have no stimulatory effect in the relatively low doses used. Whilst pseudoephedrine lacked any stimulatory effect even at supratherapeutic doses (180 mg), ephedrine possessed a stimulatory effect at therapeutic doses. Nevertheless, according to Wadler and Mainline, ephedrines exhibit less central stimulatory effects than amphetamines because they are less lipid soluble. Differences in central stimulation are related to differences of lipid solubility within the biological membranes and hence penetration of the blood-brain.

***Table:*** Urinary concentrations above which an IOC accredited laboratory must report results

| *Drug* | *Urinary concentration* |
|---|---|
| Salbutamol | > 100 ng/ml |
| Cathine | > 5 μg/ml |
| Ephedrine | > 10 μg/ml |
| Methylephedrine | > 10 μg/ml |
| Pseudoephedrine | > 25 μg/ml |
| Phenylpropanolamine | > 25 μg/ml |

barrier determines the ease with which these compounds gain access to central receptors.

## IOC REGULATIONS AND SYMPATHOMIMETIC AMINES

The use of sympathomimetic amines is restricted by the IOC. An IOC accredited laboratory must report results in excess. This constitutes a doping offence. Such offences carry with them the following penalties for a first offence:

- A warning;
- A fine of up to $100000;
- A suspension from competition for a period of 1 to 6 months.

Data from the last 5 years reveals a total of 205 cases of stimulant detection from the UK Sport's testing programme of which a high proportion were sympathomimetics.

Indeed, just over 50 per cent of cases were for ephedrines found commonly in OTC formulations. There have been numerous instances of positive tests for ephedrine. In the 1972 Munich Olympics, there was a positive test in ice hockey, but the more famous case from those Games was that of Rick Demont who lost his gold medal in the 400 m freestyle. Demont claimed that he had taken Marax for his asthma and had not been told that it contained ephedrine.

In 1988, eight US athletes tested positive for ephedrine prior to the Seoul Olympics. They were let off having claimed that it was contained within Ma Huang which they had taken inadvertently. In 1994, Diego Maradona was banished from the World Cup after testing positive for a cocktail of ephedrine and ephedrine-related substances. In 2000, the Russian synchronized swimmer, Maria Kisseleva, was stripped of her European duet title after testing positive. She claimed that it had been given to her by a team doctor to help her lose weight.

There have also been high profile cases that have involved positive tests for pseudoephedrine. In 1988 at the Seoul Olympics, the UK and subsequent Olympic 100 m champion, Linford Christie tested positive for pseudoephedrine. He was exonerated as he was believed to have taken the drug inadvertently as an ingredient of the Chinese health supplement, ginseng. What is more, although he had finished in the bronze medal position, he received the silver medal because Ben Johnson was stripped of his gold medal for using stanozolol. More recently the IOC have shown less leniency as Andreea Raducan, the Romanian gymnast was stripped of her individual gold medal at the Sydney Olympic Games after testing positive for pseudoephedrine, contained in a cold cure prescribed by the team doctor. There was an unsuccessful appeal by Raducan. Although she lost her gold medal she did not receive a ban. The doctor was less fortunate in that respect and was banned from the next two Olympiads by the IOC. The most recent example of a positive test for a respiratory drug was that of Alain Baxter at the 2002 Winter Olympics in Salt Lake City.

Alain Baxter won a bronze medal in the men's slalom but subsequently tested positive for methamphetamine. The IOC stripped Baxter of his medal. Baxter contested that he had taken the methamphetamine inadvertently by using a nasal decongestant, Vicks Inhaler. The medicine sold over-the-counter in the UK contains menthol as the active ingredient whilst that sold in the US contains methamphetamine. What is of greater significance is that the methamphetamine in the Vicks Inhaler is the l-isomer (i.e. l-methamphetamine). It is the d-isomer (d-methamphetamine) which is known colloquially as 'speed' and which has greater abuse potential because it is a central nervous system stimulant. However, the IOC test does not distinguish between the two isomers. The British Olympic Association asked the IOC to carry out the differential test but IOC President, Jacques Rogge, refused to re-open the investigation.

The International Ski Federation (FIS), who ruled that Baxter had not intentionally sought to enhance his performance, subsequently suspended Baxter for three months for the first offence of unintentionally using a prohibited substance. Baxter successfully appealed to the Court of Arbitration in Sport at Lausanne who brought forward the termination of his suspension from 15 December 2002 to 18

August 2002. However, the Court of Arbitration in Sport later rejected his appeal against disqualification by the IOC and his bronze medal was not returned. On 27 September 2002, the IOC issued a revised Prohibited List of Substances and Prohibited Methods for implementation, effective from 1 January 2003.

Included explicitly amongst several revisions were both the L- and D- isomers of the prohibited substances referred to in both Class 1.A.a. and Class 1.A.b. stimulants. There have been two less high profile cases of positive tests for ephedrines in the Olympics. There were positive tests for norephedrine (phenylpropanolamine) in yachting in Montreal followed by one in athletics in Barcelona.

In an attempt to reduce the number of positive cases and limit those athletes using sympathomimetics for legitimate reasons, the IOC introduced quantitative levels below which drug detection would not be deemed to be a positive case. It is evident that such measures are futile since pharmacokinetic data suggests that such levels are exceeded following normal therapeutic dosing.

Data from a study by Chester showed urine drug levels to remain above the IOC limits for both pseudoephedrine and phenylpropanolamine following multiple therapeutic dosing (i.e. six 60-mg doses of pseudoephedrine and six 25-mg doses of phenylpropanolamine over a 36-hour period). Drug urine concentrations were found to remain above IOC limits for a minimum of 16 hours following final administration of pseudoephedrine and a minimum of 6 hours following final administration of phenylpropanolamine.

According to the IOC, following the detection of both norpseudoephedrine and the parent compound pseudoephedrine in urine, concentrations are added in order to gain an indication of drug misuse.

It is apparent that no clear relationship exists between the amount of drug ingested and a single urine drug concentration. Indeed, drug elimination and thus urinary drug concentration are affected by several factors, including diet and activity level, all of which have an effect on urine pH and urine flow rate.

Noakes and Gillies found significant increases in urinary pseudoephedrine concentration following endurance exercise and concluded that exercise had a large but variable effect on drug elimination. The elimination of such drugs is significantly influenced by the pH of urine because basic drugs, such as sympathomimetic amines, are excreted more rapidly if urinary pH is acidic and retained in the body for longer if the urinary pH is more alkaline. Information regarding the pharmacokinetics of particular drugs is therefore essential if drug testing is to be successful in differentiating between deliberate and inadvertent drug use.

## REPUTED ERGOGENIC EFFECTS

The sympathetic response involves a myriad of reactions that heighten the capacity of the body to respond to stressful situations. Such responses include increased cardiac activity, bronchodilation, increased oxygen uptake and ventilation, redistribution of blood flow to the working muscles and increased glycogenolysis and free fatty acid mobilization. Stimulation of the central nervous system also results in an elevation in mood, an increased alertness and decreased fatigue. These actions enable an individual to perform physical activity and relate to an increased potential in terms of sports performance.

Amphetamines are structurally related to the OTC sympathomimetics and are possibly the most well known of stimulants banned by the IOC. Enhanced performance following amphetamine administration may be explained by the fact that amphetamines appear to mask the body's symptoms of fatigue. Recent data show that amphetamines are a relatively minor drug of abuse in sport these days. Ephedrines, which are much more frequently abused, are banned by the IOC because of their chemical similarity to amphetamines. Therefore, it is assumed that they, like amphetamine, have ergogenic properties. However, the literature regarding the effects of ephedrines on sports performance is limited.

Studies of the effects of sympathomimetics during exercise

can be divided into two distinct areas: those that have investigated their effects either during sub-maximal exercise or during maximal exercise.

Few studies have examined the effects of OTC stimulants on steady-state exercise. Bright et al. investigated the effects of pseudoephedrine on sub-maximal treadmill exercise. They concluded that pseudoephedrine in single or double therapeutic doses failed to cause significant cardiovascular and metabolic adjustments in healthy subjects during sub-maximal exercise. It was likely that any sympathoadrenergic effects which occurred as a result of drug administration were masked during exercise.

Most research that has attempted to elucidate the effects of such drugs on exercise has focused on performance parameters. One of the most appropriate physiological indicators of physical endurance capacity is maximal oxygen consumption (VO2max). An increase in this parameter following drug administration may indicate increased aerobic power and the potential to enhance aerobic exercise performance. Swain et al. reported no effect of pseudoephedrine and phenylpropanolamine on maximal aerobic capacity following the administration of single or double the therapeutic dose.

Similarly, Sidney and Lefcoe found no effect of a therapeutic dose of ephedrine on VO2max. demons and Crosby examined the effect of a single 60-mg dose of pseudoephedrine prior to performance of a graded exercise test and found no difference in total exercise time to exhaustion. Gillies et al. administered double the therapeutic dose of pseudoephedrine to male cyclists prior to both a 40-km time trial performed on a cycle ergometer and to a knee extension exercise. No significant effect was found either to cycling performance time or to knee extension strength. Voelz et al. investigated the effects of supratherapeutic doses of ephedrine on high intensity treadmill exercise.

There was no effect on time to exhaustion, suggesting ephedrine has no ergogenic effect even at high doses on endurance exercise. Of those studies addressing the performance effects of ephedrines, very few have used highly trained individuals or attempted to simulate competitive events.

Conduction of simple motor tasks is also an important contributing factor in athletic performance. Despite no reported ergogenic effects of OTC sympathomimetic amines upon complex exercise performance, it is possible that effects may be evident upon less complex athletic parameters such as isometric muscle strength and reaction time. However, Sidney and Lefcoe found no effect of a single therapeutic dose of ephedrine on grip strength or endurance, muscle power, anaerobic capacity or reaction time. Following multiple therapeutic doses of pseudoephedrine (i.e. six 60-mg doses over a 36-hour period) and phenylpropanolamine (six 25-mg doses over a 36-hour period) Chester found no effect on isometric grip, leg and back strength or reaction time.

Danger during endurance exercise has been associated with impaired thermoregulation as a result of the use of sympathomimetic amines. Indeed, the deaths of several cyclists during major competition, most notably that of Tom Simpson on Mont Ventoux in the 1967 Tour de France, have been attributed to hyperthermia related to the use of amphetamine. It is likely that hyperthermia is a consequence of increased motor activity and impaired thermoregulation. Although published studies have identified increased thermogenesis and a reduction in the drop in core temperature during exposure to low temperature following administration of ephedrine, no studies have assessed body temperature at comfortable ambient temperatures following the administration of ephedrines.

The use of ephedrines in sport has sometimes been associated with simultaneous use of caffeine. Bell and colleagues investigated the time to exhaustion during high intensity cycling exercise following ingestion of such a combination of drugs (5 mg/kg body weight caffeine and 1 mg/kg body weight ephedrine). Results showed a significant increase in time to exhaustion when compared with trials following placebo ingestion and ingestion of caffeine and ephedrine alone. These results were attributed to increased central nervous system stimulation. Caffeine, per se, is suspected of widespread abuse in sport. Caffeine is prohibited if the urine concentration exceeds 12 μg/ml. There was a single positive test for caffeine in the modern pentathlon in the Seoul Olympics. There is strong anecdotal evidence of caffeine abuse in cycling. In response to a questionnaire, all 12 'A' grade cyclists in a National series race in Australia reported taking caffeine before the race.

Six reported taking caffeine both before and during the race. All caffeine ingested during the race was taken within 35-50 km of the finish. The most outrageous example of simultaneous use of caffeine and other stimulants is the legendary 'pot belge'. This is a concoction purportedly used in the not-too-distant past by some cyclists and which is alleged to contain amphetamines, caffeine, cocaine, heroin, painkillers and, sometimes, corticosteroids. At least the corticosteroids are not used all the time!

The proposal that ingestion of sympathomimetic drugs can promote weight loss by increasing energy expenditure and reducing food intake through appetite suppression has resulted in considerable interest by researchers. In an animal study performed by Ramsey et al., it was reported that energy expenditure was increased and, in some animals, food intake was reduced following the administration of ephedrine and caffeine.

Consequently it was concluded that ephedrine and caffeine treatment could promote weight loss. It appears that ephedrine is effective in increasing thermogenesis and has the potential for body weight loss in obese individuals especially when combined with caffeine or aspirin. However, there have been no studies that have focused on sympathomimetic drug use and non-obese, athletic populations to promote leanness.

The number of OTC preparations which contain banned sympathomimetics is extremely high. In the USA there are over 120 formulations that contain prohibited decongestants, 36 of which contain PPA. In the UK there are over 40 formulations that contain prohibited decongestants, 11 of which contain

PPA. Moreover, even the names of products can confuse the purchaser. Thus the name Sudafed™ is associated with pseudoephedrine. But Sudafed™ tablets contain pseudoephedrine which is prohibited whilst Sudafed™ Nasal Spray contains oxymetazoline which is permitted.

## Expectorants

These are intended to increase the volume and decrease the viscosity of respiratory mucus. They are emetics, i.e. they cause vomiting at high concentrations. At sub-emetic doses they are thought to irritate the gastric mucosa, which in turn stimulates secretion of respiratory mucus by a vagal reflex, though there is little evidence to support this theory. Moreover, there is little evidence to suggest that OTC expectorants are effective. Consequently, they are frequently dismissed as little more than harmless placebos.

Guaiphenesin (guaifenesin) is the only expectorant listed by the FDA as having scientific evidence of safety and efficacy. Thick tenacious mucus that cannot be cleared by coughing is normally a feature of a bacterial infection of the lower respiratory tract rather than of a self-limiting, viral infection of the upper respiratory tract. As such, this condition may require antibiotic therapy. An alternative approach is to decrease the viscosity of mucus with a mucolytic. Steam is an excellent expectorant and mucolytic. It is permitted by the IOC and is a most acceptable alternative to the aforementioned expectorants.

## Demulcents

Demulcents substitute for the natural function of the mucus, i.e. a physical and chemical barrier which coats and protects the epithelium of the respiratory tract. Viral infections of the URT damage the epithelial lining of the respiratory tract. This reduces the production of mucus, decreases the ciliated cells which transport the mucus and reduces the protective barrier above the inflamed mucosa. A persistent, non-productive cough exacerbates the removal of cells from the respiratory epithelium and should be prevented. Demulcents are often effective in preventing dry, non-productive coughs merely by coating the inflamed tissue and protecting the exposed sensory nerve endings which initiate the cough reflex. Throat lozenges which contain a local anaesthetic (benzocaine) may be advantageous in these circumstances. Alternatively, simple linctus, syrups and lozenges containing glycerin (glycerol), honey and lemon are widely available. Note that demulcents and local anaesthetics are only effective in those areas of the URT that they can reach, i.e. the oral pharynx and larynx. However, they are often all that is needed to treat a dry, non-productive cough caused by a self-limiting viral infection and they have no side-effects. In that respect, they are preferable to centrally acting cough suppressants. Their use is permitted by the IOC.

### Xanthines

Caffeine and theophylline are methylxanthines. In the UK, seven OTC cough and cold preparations contain caffeine and three contain theophylline. One preparation even contains ephedrine in addition to both caffeine and theophylline. Theophylline is a bronchodilator which is used in Step 4 of the BTS Guidelines for the treatment of chronic asthma in adults. Caffeine is a central nervous stimulant with weak diuretic activity and little or no bronchodilator activity. Bronchodilators are of no relevance to the treatment of a congested nasal cavity, pharynx, larynx or trachea.

Bronchodilators would only be appropriate for lower respiratory tract infections where there is bronchoconstriction or a wheeze. However, in these circumstances, the presence of a cough may well be a symptom of poorly controlled asthma when the use of an OTC preparation containing a xanthine would be entirely inappropriate. Since caffeine is prohibited by the IOC when the urine concentration exceeds 12 μg/ml, there can be no justification, whatsoever, for recommending a preparation containing a xanthine to a sportsperson.

### Recommendations for Treatment of Coughs and Colds

In view of the myriad of problems facing the sportsperson

who seeks a short-term remedy for the symptoms of a cough or cold, the following recommendations are offered:

- Hydration. This will prevent dehydration when there is copious secretion and will aid expectoration when a cough is non-productive.
- Since a cough is designed to remove mucus, a productive cough should never be suppressed. A cough should only be suppressed when it is dry and non-productive (often a prelude to a viral infection of the upper respiratory tract). However, demulcents are preferable to cough suppressants if the cause is an inflamed throat because they have no side-effects and they are not banned by the IOC.
- A purulent secretion requires antibiotic therapy from a medical practitioner.
- Many cough and cold remedies cannot be recommended because they contain irrational combinations of either cough suppressants and expectorants, expectorants and antihistamines, decongestants and expectorants. Some compound preparations contain sub-therapeutic concentrations of the active ingredients. Many of the active constituents are banned by the IOC. Therefore, always attempt to purchase a product with a single active constituent. Moreover, it is cheaper to purchase an analgesic and a decongestant separately than to purchase them together in a cough and cold preparation.
- If a decongestant is desired, then caution must be applied. A topical nasal spray is always preferable as it is targeted at the desired site of action and will not have systemic side-effects. Oxymetazoline and xylometazoline are long-acting decongestants which are available as topical formulations. They need only be administered 2 and 3 times a day, respectively. Oxymetazoline, xylometazoline and phenylephrine (when administered topically) are permitted by the IOC.

- Finally, always check the list of active drugs in the pharmaceutical preparation against the list of banned drugs that is readily available. If in doubt about either the mode of action or the type of drug and whether it is likely to be banned, ask a pharmacist and then your coach. Sportspersons should heed the following emboldened warning from the IOC

Historically, the treatment of asthma and the common cold has resulted in positive drug tests and personal tragedies in the lives of elite sportspersons from Rick Demont to Andreea Raducan. As the lack of action taken against the positive tests for salbutamol and terbutaline showed in the 2000 Summer Olympiad in Sydney, it is possible to be treated for asthma and to remain within the proscribed limits set by the IOC. However, this is manifestly not the case with ephedrines when used to treat the common cold.

It would seem that routine, recommended pharmacotherapy with standard OTC cold remedies will result in urinary levels of either pseudoephedrine or phenylpropanolamine which are in excess of those laid down by the IOC, i.e. a positive drug test. Whilst this might deny a sportsperson the legitimate use of an OTC medication for a minor ailment, they would be well advised to avoid all such medications until such time as the IOC reviews the acceptable urinary concentrations of these sympathomimetics.

This does not mean that all treatments are denied them; rather, that individual medicines such as a permitted analgesic, e.g. paracetamol, and a topical decongestant, e.g. oxymetazoline, constitute a much wiser course of action and one that is not likely to end in tragedy after many years of preparation and sacrifice.

## Chapter 5

# Androgenic Anabolic Steroids

The conclusions reached in surveying anabolic steroid use in male and female athletes are that anabolic steroids do increase muscle bulk and body weight in all anabolic steroid takers but that increases in strength are certain to occur at low doses only in those undertaking regular training exercise. The long-term side-effects of anabolic steroids may be severe and will depend on dosage and duration.

In particular, early death from cardiovascular disease, sterility in men and, in women, masculinization and possible fetal effects constitute the most serious hazards. More recently, studies have suggested that psychological and behavioural changes and addiction may result from chronic anabolic steroid abuse, but methodological inconsistencies still make evaluation of these side-effects very difficult. There is evidence of increased abuse of steroids for cosmetic reasons, and among college and school students and that intensive education programmes have had little effect on steroid abuse so far.

Gliding, racialism, Jesse Owens, anabolic steroids-which is the odd one out? Well, the first three were present at the infamous Berlin Olympics of 1936, and the last one almost certainly wasn't. So when did they first make their appearance in sport? It is suggested that the Helsinki Olympics of 1952 was the debut for anabolic steroids and steroid-filled Russians then swept to numerous golds in the 1954 Vienna Weightlifting Championships. The worried US team doctor, John Ziegler, identified anabolic steroids as the source of Russian success. Armed with the new wonder drugs, the coaches, like Goethe's Sorcerer's Apprentice, wreaked a spell on their athletes, but the Sorcerer is yet to return. For centuries, it was popularly believed that symptoms of ageing in men were caused by testicular failure. This stimulated a search for an active principle of the testicles which, when isolated, would restore sexual and mental vigour to ageing men. The testicular principle, we now know, is the male sex hormone testosterone, which was first synthesized in 1935.

Experimental studies in both animals and humans soon showed that testosterone possessed both anabolic and androgenic actions. The androgenic actions of testosterone are those actions involving the development and maintenance of primary and secondary sexual characteristics while the anabolic actions consist of the positive effects of testosterone in inhibiting urinary nitrogen loss and stimulating protein synthesis, particularly in skeletal muscle.

## THE TESTOSTERONE FAMILY

Testosterone is a so-called C-19 steroid hormone. The steroid hormones are derived in the body from the substance cholesterol. The structure of testosterone is closely related to the steroid substance androstane and the structure of androstane is used as a reference when naming most of the compounds related to or derived from testosterone. The apparently identical structures of testosterone and epitestosterone can be differentiated by the orientation of the hydrogen atom at the 17 position. When two chemical compounds have the same atomic composition, but different orientations of the constituent atoms, they are known as isomers. Hence epitestosterone is an isomer of testosterone.

### Biosynthesis

In humans, the immediate precursor of testosterone in the biosynthetic sequence from cholesterol is androstenedione which is converted to testosterone by the action of the enzyme 17b-hydroxysteroid dehydrogenase. This enzyme will also act on other steroids with similar structures, such as 19 nor-androstenedione, to produce 19 nor-testosterone (nandrolone).

## THE BIOCHEMISTRY AND PHYSIOLOGY OF TESTOSTERONE

Testosterone, the most important naturally occurring compound with androgen and anabolic activity is formed in the Leydig cells of the testis but also in the adrenal cortex.

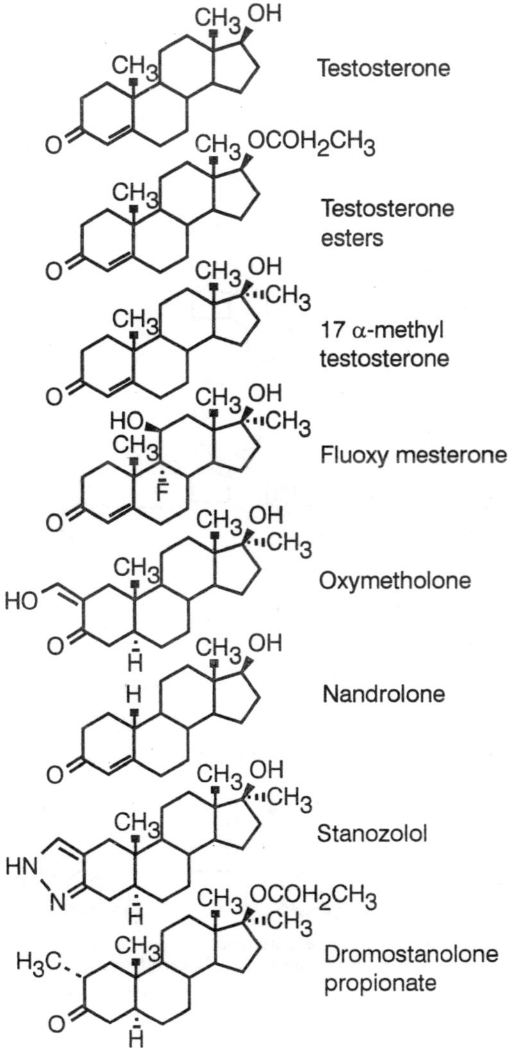


**Fig.** The Structure of Testosterone

Adrenocortical testosterone is important in women, as it is responsible for some secondary sexual characteristics such as pubic and axillary hair growth and in some cases for its influence on sexuality. Mean testosterone production in men is approximately 8 mg per day of which 90-95 per cent is produced by the testis and the remainder by the adrenal cortex. When testosterone is synthesized in the body, its isomer epitestosterone is also formed. Epitestosterone has exactly the same number of atoms as testosterone but the "H and "OH groups at C-17 are orientated differently.

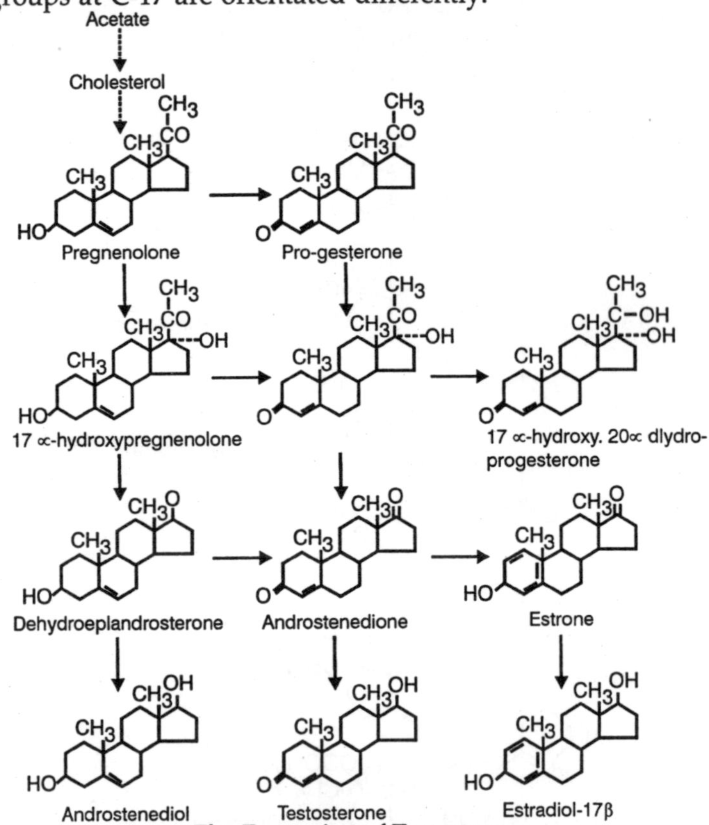


**Fig.** Formation of Testosterone

The ratio of testosterone to epitesterone concentrations in the plasma of normal males is 12:1. The testis also produces 5a-dihydrotestosterone, which is approximately equal in androgenic and anabolic activity to testosterone, and also two compounds with much weaker biological activity: androstenedione and dehydroepian-drosterone. After puberty, plasma testosterone levels are approximately 0.6 mg/dl in males and 0.03 mg/dl in women; 95 per cent of testosterone in the blood is bound to protein, mainly sex hormone-binding globulin (SHBG); 2-3 per cent of testosterone remains free, i.e. unbound, while the remainder is bound to serum albumin.

## MODE OF ACTION OF TESTOSTERONE

Like most other steroid hormones testosterone produces its principal effect on tissues by altering cellular biochemistry via an interaction with the cell nucleus. Testosterone diffuses into the cell, as it is lipid soluble and thus readily crosses cell membranes.

It combines with a testosterone-binding protein which transports it to the cell nucleus. Here the testosterone interacts on a particular chromosome with one or more specific binding sites called hormone receptor elements and activates the synthesis of one or more proteins which may be either enzymes or structural proteins.

However, the possibility that testosterone and/or anabolic steroids may produce pharmacological effects via a cell surface receptor should not be ruled out. In some mammalian tissues such cell surface receptors are known to exist for the glucocorticoid hormones, which also possess a similar steroid structure to testosterone. In some tissues testosterone is first converted to 5α-dihydrotestosterone (DHT), also called androstanolone, by the enzyme 5α-reductase. The DHT is then transported to the nucleus and produces similar biochemical changes to those of testosterone.

In many testosterone-sensitive tissues it is now thought that the anabolic effects of testosterone are mainly produced by the action of DHT. DHT can be formed from testosterone in the testes, liver, brain, prostate gland and external genitalia, but there is little 5α-reductase activity and therefore little direct formation of DHT in human skeletal muscle. Generally in the liver, and locally in brain areas such as the hypothalamus, testosterone can be converted by the aromatase enzyme system to oestradiol.

The 'aromatization' of testosterone to oestradiol is essential for sexual differentiation of the brain, bone mass consolidation and for epiphyseal fusion of the long bones at the end of puberty. DHT is primarily androgenic while oestradiol antagonizes some androgenic actions while enhancing others. The full details of testosterone synthesis and metabolism have been expertly reviewed by Wilson, Lukas, Wu, and Ueki and Okana.

## Metabolism

Apart from conversion to DHT in various tissues, testosterone is metabolized in the liver mainly to DHT, androstenedione and then via the 3-keto reductive enzymes to either androsterone or one of its two isomers, epiandrosterone or etiocholanolone.

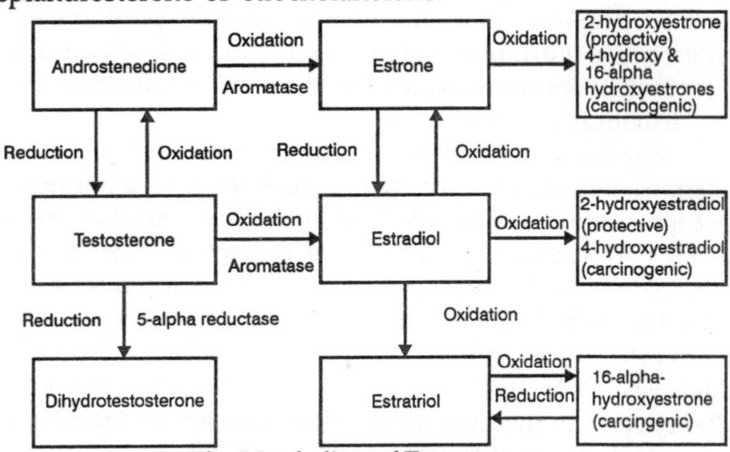


**Fig.** Metabolism of Testosterone

This has been reviewed recently by Ueki and Okana and Wright et al.. All four metabolites are present in plasma and urine. Androsterone and epiandrosterone have weak androgenic activity, while etiocholanone has none.

Some testosterone is converted in the testis to oestradiol. Significant amounts of oestradiol are also thought to be formed from testosterone in the brain.

## Androgenic Effects

Testosterone is responsible for the development of primary sexual characteristics in males. Normally in a genetically male fetus, i.e. one with the XY sex chromosome configuration, the embryonic testis begins to differentiate, under the influence of H-Y antigen, the production of which is directed by the Y chromosome. As the male gonad differentiates, Leydig cells are formed which begin to secrete testosterone. Testosterone and a polypeptide factor Müllerian regression factor (MRF) together stimulate the formation of the internal male genitalia, in utero. The external genitalia and prostate develop mainly under the influence of DHT. From birth until puberty the Leydig cells which secrete testosterone produce small amounts of testosterone providing a plasma testosterone concentration of up to 2 nmol/. From the age of approximately 10 years, in males, increased testosterone secretion occurs principally from the testicular Leydig cells.

The pubertal changes induced by this increase in testosterone are the secondary sexual characteristics which include musculoskeletal configuration, genital size, psychic changes and induction of sperm production. Adult secondary hair growth is stimulated by DHT. The chronology of male puberty and adolescence has been described in detail by Tanner and the Tanner Index provides a useful guide for the assessment of the progress of puberty, and the attainment of maturity.

## Anabolic Effects

The anabolic effects of testosterone and anabolic steroids are usually considered to be those promoting protein synthesis and muscle growth, but they also include effects such as stimulation and eventually inhibition of skeletal growth in the young. Attempts to produce purely anabolic, synthetic, testosterone derivatives have been unsuccessful. It should be remembered that though the anabolic action of anabolic steroids may be much greater than testosterone, all anabolic steroids also possess some androgenic activity. There will also be discrete variations in the ratio of androgenic to anabolic activity amongst the family of testosterone derivatives, anabolic steroids and their various metabolites. For example, it has been suggested that, in females, the androgenic effect of the nandrolone metabolite 19 nor-dihydro-testosterone.

## STRUCTURAL ANALOGUES OF TESTOSTERONE-THE ANABOLIC STEROIDS

To the dismay of clinical scientists, it was soon discovered that when the newly isolated testosterone was given orally or injected into patients it was ineffective. When taken by mouth, testosterone is absorbed from the small intestine and passes via the portal vein to the liver where it is rapidly metabolized, mostly to inactive compounds. Injected testosterone also passes rapidly into the blood and then to the liver where it is inactivated. In the late 1940s medicinal chemists began to develop analogues of testosterone which might be degraded less easily by the body. Forty years of intensive research have yielded three major types of testosterone modification, each of which gives rise to a class of anabolic steroids.

Addition of an alkyl group at position 17 renders the structure orally inactive (B). A type (A) modification makes the compound suitable for 'depot' injection, while type (C) modifications allow oral dosing and sometimes increased potency. A detailed account of the medicinal chemistry of anabolic steroids is provided by Wilson while a brief introduction to the topic is provided by George.

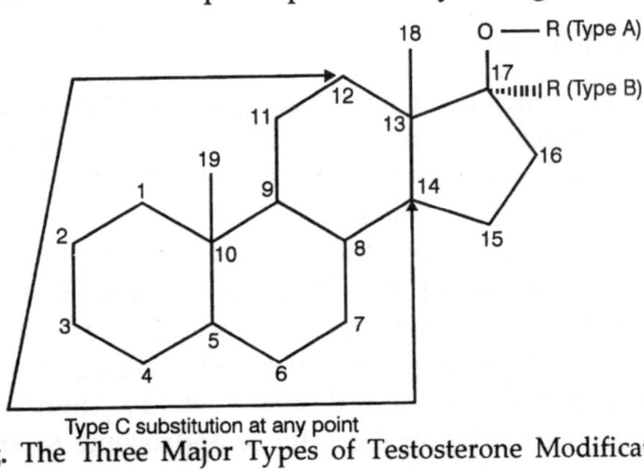


**Fig.** The Three Major Types of Testosterone Modification

## CLINICAL USES OF ANDROGENS/ANABOLIC STEROIDS

### Replacement Therapy in Men

Anabolic steroids may be given to stimulate sexual development in cases of delayed puberty. The therapy is then withdrawn gradually once full sexual maturity is reached. They may also be given in cases where the testicles have been surgically removed either because of physical injury or because of a testicular tumour. In this case the replacement therapy must be continuous for life.

### Replacement Therapy in Women

Testosterone production is necessary in women as well as men. In the rare condition known as sexual infantilism a young female fails to secrete oestradiol, progesterone and testosterone. As a consequence she suffers from amenorrhea, a lack of libido and absence of pubic and axillary hair. Only when she is treated with testosterone does libido appear. Some postmenopausal women suffer from loss of libido. In both these cases administration of testosterone restores sex drive and sexual characteristics.

### Gynaecological Disorders

Anabolic steroids are occasionally used to treat gynaecological conditions in women, though long-term usage produces severe side-effects such as erratic menstruation and the appearance of male secondary characteristics. In the USA, they have sometimes been used to repress lactation, after childbirth. They are also sometimes used to combat breast tumours in premenopausal women.

## PROTEIN ANABOLISM

The initial use of anabolic steroids in the early 1940s was to inhibit the loss of protein and aid muscle regeneration after major surgery, and to stimulate muscle regeneration in debilitating disorders such as muscular dystrophy and diabetes. Many concentration camp survivors owe their early recovery from debilitation to the skilled use of dietary measures coupled with anabolic steroids. Recently, a number of clinical studies have indicated that nandrolone, oxandrolone and oxy-methalone may be able to attenuate and, in some cases, reverse muscle loss and decline of lean body mass in AIDS patients.

## Anaemia

Anabolic steroids are sometimes used in large doses to treat anaemias which have proved resistant to other therapies-this therapy is not recommended in women because of masculinizing side-effects.

There is some evidence that combined oestrogen/androgen therapy is able to inhibit bone degeneration in this disorder. Anabolic steroids may be used to increase growth in prepubertal boys who have failed to reach their expected height for their age. The treatment must be carried out under carefully controlled conditions so that early fusion of the epiphyses does not occur.

## Side-effects of Androgens

These include acne, growth of facial hair, hoarsening or deepening of the voice and reduction in body fat. If the dose given is sufficient to suppress gonadotrophin secretion then menstrual irregularities will occur. Chronic, i.e. long-term treatment with androgens, as for example in mammary carcinoma, may produce the following side-effects-male pattern baldness, prominent musculature and veins, clitoral hypertrophy. A detailed review of this subject has been provided by Elliott and Goldberg. A case of gender identify confusion coupled with pseudohermaphroditism has been reported recently.

Administration of androgens can cause stunting of growth, a side-effect directly related to disturbance of normal bone growth and development. The enhancement of epiphyseal closure is a particularly persistent side-effect which can be present up to 3 months after androgen withdrawal. Spermatogenesis is reduced by testosterone treatment with as little as 25 mg of testosterone per day over a 6-week period. Anabolic steroids will produce the same effect, since they will suppress natural testosterone secretion. The inhibition of Spermatogenesis may persist for many months after anabolic steroid withdrawal.

## GENERAL SIDE-EFFECTS

### OEDEMA

Oedema or water retention, related to the increased retention of sodium and chloride is a frequent side-effect of short-term androgen administration. This may be the major contribution to the initial weight gain seen in athletes taking these drugs. Water and electrolyte gain is an unwanted side-effect in all normal individuals but is particularly unhealthy in people with circulatory disorders or in those with a family background of such disorders.

### BLOOD VOLUME

Significant increases in steroid-induced water retention are likely to produce an increase in the blood volume. It should be noted that any expansion of the blood volume is likely to be a result of the simultaneous increase in water retention plus the increased erythropoiesis caused by anabolic steroid administration.

### JAUNDICE

Jaundice is a frequent side-effect of anabolic steroid therapy and is caused mainly by reduced flow and retention of bile in the biliary capillaries of the hepatic lobules. Hepatic cell damage is not usually present. Those anabolic steroids with a 17α-methyl group are most likely to cause jaundice.

### HEPATIC CARCINOMA

Patients who have received androgens and/or anabolic steroids for prolonged periods may develop hepatic carcinoma. This is also particularly prevalent in people who have taken 17α-methyl testosterone derivatives.

## ANABOLIC STEROIDS AND SPORT

The desire to increase sporting performance and athletic prowess by means other than physical training has been experienced for at least 2000 years. Ryan quotes the observation of the Greeks that a high protein diet was essential for bodybuilding and athletic achievement. The Greeks, of course, knew nothing of protein structure or biosynthesis but they felt that by eating the flesh of a strong animal such as the ox, the athlete would gain strength himself. We have seen previously that one of the first therapeutic uses of anabolic steroids was in treating the protein loss and muscle wasting suffered by concentration camp victims.

Following the publication of the results of these treatments it was natural that anabolic steroids should be used in an attempt to increase muscle strength in athletes. Many early studies on the effect of anabolic steroids often involved self-administration and were necessarily anecdotal with no attempt at scientific or controlled investigation of the effect of the steroid drugs. Several studies relied on subjective feelings and lacked any objective measure of increased strength or stamina. Also, side-effects were never admitted to or were simply omitted from the results. Subsequent studies, many of which were carried out in the late 1960s and early 1970s, were more scientifically based but often entirely contradictory in their results.

### Sources, Supply and Control

The increased usage of anabolic steroids by athletes and the spread of usage from sport to the general population has prompted governmental intervention in several countries and stimulated investigation into the illicit supply of anabolic steroids and the control of their abuse.

In Great Britain, anabolic steroids are licensed by the Department of Health's Medicine Control Agency (MCA) as prescription-only medicines (POMs) within the meaning of the Medicines Act 1968. This means that it is illegal for a doctor or pharmacist to supply them other than by a doctor's prescription and there are recorded cases of individual prosecution for illegal supply. The UK government has legislated to classify anabolic steroids as controlled drugs under the Misuse of Drugs Act. This makes export, import, and supply without prescription illegal. Under UK law, possession of anabolic steroids is not illegal unless it is 'with intent to supply' whether for profit or not. This attitude has been contested by many experts on addiction and those closely associated with counselling and treating anabolic problems in gyms and sports clubs. Denmark has recently raised anabolic steroids to 'controlled' status and has made possession a criminal offence punishable by two years in jail.

In the USA anabolic steroids were added to Schedule III of the Controlled Substances Act of 1994, making supply and possession of the drugs a federal offence. However, the American Medical Association opposed this legislation because they contend that most of the illicitly used anabolic steroids are illegally smuggled in or manufactured, and such legislation, when enacted for cocaine led to an increase in its illegal supply.

There are numerous sources of anabolic steroids, which vary between nations. In the USA, the major external sources appear to be Panama and Mexico, while illegal synthesis by 'street traders' is another major source. Both these internal and external sources provide drugs which are untested, unstandardized, contain potentially toxic impurities and have not been produced in the stringently hygienic conditions of the modern pharmaceutical industry. Musshoff et al. analysed 42 illicit 'anabolic' substances seized by the police and customs officials in Germany. Fifteen of these contained counterfeit ingredients such as 'cheaper' anabolic steroids substituted for more expensive products, for example metenolone gestagen (a progestogen) substituted for nandrolone.

In two cases tocopherole (an anabolically inactive compound) was substituted for the steroid trenbolone. There are anecdotal tales of body builders taking 'anabolic steroids' which were actually stilboestrol, an oestrogen used in Europe for improving the muscle mass of chickens. Perry et al. described the supply of Equipoise, an equine anabolic steroid, to gym users in Glamorgan. Catlin et al. examined seven brands of androstenedione available 'over the counter' in US health shops and only one contained the pure compound; the others consisted of adulterated product, impurities such as testosterone and in one sample no drug at all. Surveys show that the majority of steroid abusers in the USA are supplied by the black market with the remaining supplies coming from physicians and pharmacists. In their survey of college student athletes, Green et al. found that 32 per cent of anabolic steroid abusers in the USA obtained their drugs from a physician not associated with the college team!

All these criminal activities are insignificant in terms of organization and scale compared with the sponsored and managed promotion and supply of anabolic steroids by the government of the former German Democratic Republic (GDR). Release of State documents following the GDR's collapse indicates the extent of the systematic, programmed dosing of thousands of GDR athletes in the period 1970-1990. A full account of this governmental network of drug supply and administration in the cause of athletic abuse has been provided by Franke and Berendonk. There is every reason to suppose that the practice has occurred elsewhere and is continuing.

## PATTERNS OF ADMINISTRATION AND USE

No two groups of athletes who abuse anabolic steroids seem to use the same pattern of drug administration. It is this observation that above all confounds attempts to make scientific comparisons between various studies of anabolic steroid efficacy. There are a number of administration regimes in use though each has its variations and often combinations of regimes may be used concurrently.

### Cycling

A period of administration followed by a similar period of abstinence before the administration is recommenced. Typical cycling patterns are short: 6-8 weeks on drug, 6-8 weeks' abstinence; or long: 6-18 weeks on drug with up to 12 months' abstinence. The rationale here is that the periods of abstinence may reduce the incidence of side-effects. This regime is preferred by body builders.

## Pyramiding

A variation of cycling in which the dose is gradually built up in the cycle to a peak and then gradually reduced again towards the end of the cycle. This regime is said to cause fewer behavioural side-effects such as lowered mood, caused by the withdrawal of the drug.

## Stacking

The use of more than one anabolic steroid at a time. In its simplest form this regime involves the simultaneous use of both an orally administered steroid and an injectable one. More 'sophisticated' patterns involve intricate schedules of administration using many different steroids each with supposedly different pharmacological profiles. The aim of this technique is to avoid plateauing, that is, the development of tolerance to a particular drug. According to the amateur pharmacologists of locker rooms and gymnasia, these 'super stacking' programmes allow more receptor sites to be stimulated. This is very dubious pharmacology since the number of intracellular testosterone/DHT steroid receptors is stable and all are probably saturated under normal physiological conditions.

Exact doses tried by abusers are almost impossible to establish. What is certain is that doses used by weightlifters and body builders are at least 100 times those indicated for therapeutic use and also those used in most scientific studies. The dose-response studies of Forbes also indicate that the doses used in 'ethical/clinical' studies of anabolic steroid effects on athletic performance are only sufficient to cause modest improvements in lean body mass. It is claimed that endurance and sprint athletes who abuse steroids may use doses closer to clinical recommendations.

The abuse cycles documented above are often followed in males by a dose of human chorionic gonadotrophin (hGG), which is used to stimulate endogenous testosterone production that has been suppressed by the chronic administration of testosterone or anabolic steroids.

## Extent of usage

It is difficult to calculate which anabolic steroid is most often abused world-wide. Some anabolic steroids are not available in every country, some are stolen veterinary preparations and some have been illicitly manufactured. Many athletes will also be 'stacking' several preparations at once. The most popular abused drugs in the US college survey of Pope while in a survey of US power-lifters the most popular drugs were methandrostenolone (93 per cent) and testosterone esters (80 per cent).

The first British survey of anabolic steroid usage dianabol (methandrostenolone) at 69 per cent was the most frequently administered anabolic steroid. In their study, published in 1994, Pope and Katz found that the majoirity of abusers reported taking testosterone, while 54 per cent admitted taking nandrolone. When the urine of the same athletes was tested, only 41 per cent were found to be abusing testosterone and 57 per cent nandrolone. This study illustrates the possible confusion of different drugs by abusers or the possibility of deception by drug suppliers.

| *Drug* | *No. abusing drug** |
|---|---|
| Dianabol<br>Deca Durabolin | 43<br>37 |
| Testosterone esters | 32 |
| Stanozolol | 19 |
| Equipoise | 10 |
| *More than one drug abused by some subjects. | |

In 1994, Chinese athletes were alleged to be abusing dihydrotestosterone. Later surveys have shown minor changes in drug preferences and also for the first time the most popular anabolic steroids taken by females. The 1997 UK survey carried out by Korkia and Stimson at six separate sites in the UK, showed testosterone, nandrolone and dianobol were equally popular amongst male abusers while female abusers preferred oxandiolone, stanozolol and methandrostenlone. Though only 13 women (compared with 97 men) took part in the survey, it is interesting that women seemed to prefer orally active drugs. A local survey in the Clwyd area of North Wales also found differences in anabolic steroid preferences between males and females though in this survey some women, of the eight surveyed, did use nandrolone, whereas the 62 males used three different injectable anabolic steroids and four different orally active drugs.

Data from the infamous GDR archives on the 'State' doping of athletes shows that both orally active and injectable anabolic steroids were used in their abuse programme. There is also the sinister documentation of coded, unnamed 'steroid substance' possibly indicacting that some covert evaluations/clinical trials of drugs or new products were being undertaken.

## POLYPHARMACY

The concurrent abuse of anabolic steroids with other drugs has also been a feature of surveys conducted twice since the 1980s. These additional abuses usually involve drugs taken to counteract the side-effects of anabolic steroids. In the 1992 survey 5 per cent of anabolic steroid abusers were additionally taking the anti-oestrogen tamoxifen. This was to counteract the feminizing effects produced by the conversion to oestradiol of the testosterone they were taking. Korkia and Stimson found 22.7 per cent of their abusers taking hCG, possibly for the reasons given earlier. A further 22.7 per cent were taking anti-oestrogens and 11.8 per cent were taking antibiotics, presumably to counteract acne.

Several surveys report alarming co-administration of anabolic steroids and stimulants. In their survey of US college students Meilman et al. found 44.7 per cent of steroid abusers also took amphetamine and 40.8 per cent cocaine. Both these drugs are stimulants, taken to aid weight loss or counteract negative psychological effects of steroid abuse. Diuretics are frequently co-abused with anabolic steroids and were noted in several surveys. Evans reported 22 per cent of anabolic steroid abusers in Glamorgan were taking diuretics, probably to counteract the water retention induced by anabolic steroids.

## THE EPIDEMIOLOGY OF ANABOLIC STEROID ABUSE

In response to the widespread view that anabolic steroid abuse was rife in the sporting population, several American investigators began surveys of athletes in order to establish the distribution and prevalence of anabolic steroid abuse. These useful investigations are continuing. In a summary of these early findings, Pope et al. reported that as many as 20 per cent of intercollegiate athletes and fewer than 1 per cent of non-athlete students reported using anabolic steroids. This prevalence was much higher than the 2.5 per cent usage rate reported in a 1971 study. The review by Pope et al. also records a survey of students at a Florida High School where 18 per cent of male students but no females reported using anabolic steroids.

From their own survey of 1010 college males, Pope et al. found that 2 per cent reported taking anabolic steroids, with university-standard athletes more likely to be taking steroids than non-athletes. Of this 2 per cent, 42 per cent reported that body building and appearance were their main reasons for anabolic steroid abuse; 58 per cent reported various reasons connected with sport for their abuse. High degrees of prevalence of abuse (6.6 per cent) were found by Buckley et al. in 1700 US high school students, while Windsor and Dumitru found a 3 per cent abuse level in 800 US college students. In this survey 5 per cent of males and 1.4 per cent of females admitted abusing steroids. Williamson has carried out the major British study of anabolic steroid abuse and found levels of 4.4 per cent in males, 1 per cent in females at a college of technology in Scotland.

When surveys of non-college athletes are conducted the percentage of abusers is much higher. Yesalis et al. found a current prevalence of 33 per cent amongst US powerlifters, which rose to 55 per cent when previous usage amongst non-users was included. In the UK, Perry et al. reported a 38.8 per cent prevalence amongst weight-trainers in private gymnasia in their West Glamorgan survey area.

The figures for young abusers in GB and the USA-3-6 per cent-may vary in different locations. In Britain, there is anecdotal evidence to suggest that anabolic steroid abuse is higher in areas with a macho culture, ample male leisure time (i.e. unemployment), low self-esteem and proximity to sandy beaches. Thus abuse may be said to be led by cultural pressure, feelings of social inadequacy and a suitable location to parade the results of your body-building. The high prevalence of steroid abuse in Florida (18 per cent according to Pope et al, 1988) may well reflect this latter theory! In Australia, Handelsman and Gupta found that the 3.2 per cent of high school boys who abused anabolic steroids were frequently truants.

The prevalence of anabolic steroid abuse in international competition is difficult to judge. At the 1972 (pre-testing) Munich Olympics, 68 per cent of interviewed athletes in middle or short distance running or in field events admitted taking steroids. At the Mexico Olympics, all the US weightlifters admitted taking steroids. Perhaps the introduction of mandatory testing for the 1976 Olympics in Montreal has led to a decline in steroid abuse rather than a switching to less detectable doping agents such as hGH. The official IOC figures in 2000 show that though anabolic steroid abuse at IOC accredited events as a percentage of total positive results was 38.1 per cent compared with 65.3 per cent in 1986, the actual numbers of positive anabolic steroid tests was up from 439 in 1986 to 946 in 2000. We may also have to regard the current generation of athletes as a lost cause and instead concentrate education and deterrent resources on the young. Up to 1992, progress in the USA had encouraged some experts to suggest that the availability and usage of steroids in the USA is decreasing. But analysis of the trends in the USA by Yesalis and Bahrke shows that this optimism is unfounded as the abuse figures generally are static and in some surveys may be increasing.

# EFFICACY OF ANABOLIC STEROIDS

## EFFECTS ON MUSCLE

Whether anabolic steroid treatment 'works' has been perhaps the most difficult question of all to answer satisfactorily since many of the early investigations that have been carried out were, in the main, poorly designed scientifically, clinically and statistically. Increases in muscle strength are proportional to increases in the cross-sectional diameter of the muscles being trained but there is no way of showing conclusively, in vivo, that any increase in muscle diameter consists of increased muscle protein rather than increased content of water or fat. Advances in the use of ultrasound and NMR (nuclear magnetic resonance) techniques may make this possible early in the 2000s, and some progress has been made in the analysis of the effects of exercise and drugs on muscle structure.

It is also apparent that different groups of athletes may wish to increase their muscle bulk for different purposes. For example, the American footballer or the wrestler may wish simply to increase his bulk and weight, whereas a weightlifter may want increased dynamic strength and the long distance runner may wish to accelerate muscle repair after an arduous and taxing run.

The first serious investigator of the question as to whether anabolic steroids work seems to be Ryan who reviewed a total of 37 studies between the years 1968 and 1977. He was confounded by the many different measurements being taken as indices of anabolic steroid activity. Some studies attempted to measure gains in strength of experimental subjects over controls, other studies measured the change in circumference of a limb. One study attempted to measure change in lean body mass. In 12 studies which claimed that athletes taking anabolic steroids gained in strength, the gains reported were often quite small. The majority of these 12 studies were not 'blind': that is either the investigator or the subject (or perhaps both!) knew when an active principle was being taken. In only five of the studies were protein supplements given and in none of the studies examined was there any dietary control or at least a listing of total protein and caloric intake for each subject. Other features of these studies were their poor design in matching control and experimental subjects and there were also errors in calculating the results.

Ryan then examined 13 other studies in which valid matching of controls and experiments had occurred. Ten of these 13 studies were double blind (neither experimenter or subject knew when an active substance was being administered), the control and experimental groups contained at least six subjects in each and the average period of experimentation was some 50 per cent longer than in the early studies in which improvements were claimed. Also, in this second group of experiments, five different steroid groups were investigated compared with only two in the earlier group. Ryan's conclusion from examining these two groups of studies was that there was no substantial evidence for an increase in lean muscle bulk or muscle strength in healthy young adult males receiving anabolic steroids.

Comparison of these studies is difficult because the various parameters used to assess improvement in strength were not the same. Though the majority of studies assessed by Ryan measured changes in gross body weight and 'improvement' in standard strength tests, the other tests employed included VO2max, limb circumference, lean body mass and 'changes in blood chemistry'. One reason for the variety of measurements used and a possible explanation for the lack of agreement in assessing anabolic steroid efficacy is that different athletic groups each sought different parameters for improvement. As I have mentioned before, the American footballer or wrestler may be seeking increased bulk, the weightlifter or thrower an increase in strength or perhaps both.

Experiments with anabolic steroids, since 1975, have tended to be more carefully carried out, controlled and more sophisticated than those reviewed by Ryan. An example of an early, well-conducted trial is the frequently quoted study by Freed et al.. In this experiment six standard strength exercises were used as a measure of increased strength. The study was carried out over a 6-week period in weightlifters who were given either 10 or 25 mg per day of methandienone. Drug treatment increased strength by 0.3-13 per cent during the 6-week study while those taking placebo showed strength gains of 0.3-2.3 per cent. Body weight increased only in the drug-treated athletes and those on the 25 mg dose showed no greater strength increase than those on 10 mg.

A significant finding was that withdrawal of the anabolic steroid caused a loss of weight but no loss in strength gained, which suggested that anabolic steroid taking amongst athletes might be harder to detect since the drug could be withdrawn from an athlete well in advance of a meeting without significant loss of performance, thus allowing him to evade detection in any doping test. Further analysis of Freed's study shows that the doses of methandienone are some 75 per cent lower than those claimed to be used by some athletes.

It might have been more useful to tailor the dose of the drug to the athlete's initial body weight, i.e. calculate the dose in terms of mg/kg body weight, and also to measure the actual free and bound plasma concentration of the drug. It is reasonable to conclude from Freed's work that only a proportion of people show a significant improvement in strength as a result of steroid treatment.

Studies should also determine who are the types of athlete or individual which 'benefit' from anabolic steroids. Another factor absent from the analyses of this and other earlier experiments is consideration of the subject's body build. The bodily changes induced by testosterone at puberty and indeed those that are produced in utero occur as a result of an interaction between testosterone and the individual genetic 'constitution' or genotype.

Thus, the individual emerging from puberty with a lean, well-muscled body-the classic mesomorph somatotype-does so because of the expression of the genes controlling his muscularity rather than because he has higher testosterone levels than the more lightly muscled ectomorph. Thus, only certain somatotypes may benefit fully An important early study on the influence of athletic experience and pre-training on the response of athletes to anabolic steroid treatment was researched by Wright. He noted that inexperienced weightlifters showed no increase in strength or lean muscle mass while simultaneously taking anabolic steroids and protein supplements and undergoing short-term training. In contrast, weightlifters who trained regularly, i.e. to nearly their maximum capacity, did show increased strength compared with their pretreatment level.

Though his results did not show consistent increases in strength amongst the steroid-treated trained athletes, Wright claimed to show that the trained athletes responded better to anabolic steroid treatment, a finding he could not explain adequately. However, the presence of a greater initial muscle mass in the trained athletes before anabolic steroid treatment might have been a factor. Another possibility is that trained muscles are different, i.e. they may produce some endogenous factor which enhances anabolic steroid action. It is already known that the muscles of trained athletes can increase their uptake of glucose by the production of an endogenous factor and that regular exercise regimes increase the responsiveness of skeletal muscle to insulin.

If the results of these studies, from 20 years ago, produce such inconsistent results, why do athletes continue to take anabolic steroids? One possible explanation was that the steroid trials so far are based on dose levels which, while medically and ethically acceptable, are considerably less than those commonly taken by athletes. This factor coupled with the necessity of pre-drug intensive training and a high protein diet might explain the failure of anabolic steroids to produce a consistent increase in strength and performance.

The importance of training during and before a period of steroid treatment is apparently emphasized in a sophisticated series of experiments carried out by Hervey and colleagues between 1976 and 1981, and reviewed by Hervey. The experimental design involved the administration of the anabolic steroid dianabol at 100 mg per day during one 6-week period and a placebo during the other 6 weeks. The two treatment periods (drug and placebo) were separated by a 6-

week treatment-free period. The experiments were carried out double blind. All volunteers were athletes, one group being professional weightlifters. In each group, body weight, body fat, body density and the fat and lean tissue proportion were measured.

The non-weightlifting group of athletes showed the same improvement in weightlifting performance and leg muscle strength during both placebo and drug administration periods. In the group containing experienced weightlifters there was a significant improvement during drug administration when compared with the placebo period. Both weightlifters and other athletes exhibited weight gain and increases in limb circumference. Though the weightlifters were heavier than their non-weightlifting counterparts, the proportion of lean body mass was the same in both groups.

Hervey et al. concluded from these experiments that in athletes engaged in continuous hard-training regimes, anabolic steroids in the doses athletes claim to use cause an increase in muscle strength and athletic performance. The experimental design could be criticized in that it is possible that those subjects taking the drug in the first 6-week period were not completely drug free at the start of the placebo period 6 weeks later. Thus, the residual effect of the steroid could have affected measurements during the placebo period of evaluation and could have masked any apparent difference between the placebo and treatment periods.

These are two examples of well-conducted trials carried out in the early 1980s. Summarizing the evidence gained from these and earlier trials, Haupt and Rovere concluded that abuse of anabolic steroids will consistently result in a significant increase in strength if all of the following criteria are satisfied.

- They are given to athletes who have been intensively trained in weightlifting immediately before the start of the steroid regimen and who continue this intensive weightlift training during the steroid regimen.
- The athletes maintain a high protein diet.

- The changes in the athletes' strength are measured by the single repetition/ maximal weight technique for those exercises with which the athlete trains.

Studies demonstrating significant increases in body size and body weight during the anabolic steroid regimen were consistently those studies that demonstrated statistically significant increases in strength.

Studies that did not demonstrate significant increases in body size and body weight during the anabolic steroid regimen were consistently those studies that did not demonstrate statistically significant increases in strength.

Janet Elashoff and her colleagues at Cedars Sinai Medical Centre, Los Angeles have provided an even more sophisticated analysis of 30 of these early studies in which athletes received two or more doses of anabolic steroid and in which changes in muscular strength were measured. They made use of the statistical technique known as meta-analysis and also analysed for the statistical power of the study. In addition to the study defects described previously, Elashoff et al. found marked evidence of poor statistical design and computation in many of the 30 studies examined; for example, the use of standard instead of paired t tests when comparing paired data.

They queried whether any of the studies were truly blind and whether checks for compliance were carried out properly. Their conclusions were that, in many cases, it must be obvious to both experimenter and athlete who is on an active preparation since it should be possible to see who develops greater acne, beard growth and weight gain and the athletes will almost certainly experience the psychopharmacological effects of 'being on steroids'.

As in previous reviews the authors question whether further analysis of these studies is worthwhile since the amounts administered are obviously below the amounts used by the abusing adult. Referring to the studies of Forbes quoted previously, it is obvious that the maximum dose of 7245 mg used in the experiments reviewed by Elashoff is at the start of the drug dose/lean body mass curve and thus only just at the threshold of producing an observable improvement in lean body mass. The latest research seems to confirm that supraphysiological doses of anabolic steroids do have effects over and above low doses used in earlier studies.

In his 1997 computation of testosterone doses in relation to plasma level, Wu suggested that the responses to anabolic steroids obtained at the supraphysiological doses and plasma levels used by many abusers were part of a different/separate relationship than that obtained to physiological or clinical plasma levels. He doubted whether results obtained at ethical/clinical levels of dosage could be extrapolated to the high dosage levels used by many abusers. A year previously, Bhasin et al. designed a study incorporating many of the suggestions made by earlier reviewers.

This well-controlled study recruited 43 volunteers and compared supraphysiological testosterone doses with placebo, with or without exercise, over a 10-week period. The dosing regime of the treated subjects was a 6000 mg injection of testosterone enanthrate per week. There was a strictly controlled exercise and dietary regime. Results showed an increase in muscle strength with exercise alone. Testosterone alone increased muscle size, strength and lean body mass, but each of these values could be increased further by simultaneous exercise. Supraphysiological doses of testosterone, and presumably also other androgens, according to this vital study do have an anabolic effect on muscle mass, strength and lean body mass in men and this can be enhanced by physical training regimes.

In a later review of his own and other studies, Bhasin et al. concluded that testosterone supplementation increases maximal voluntary strength but that it does not improve specific tension. Thus testosterone would be expected to improve performance in weightlifting events as these activities are so dependent on maximal voluntary strength. No studies have yet demonstrated any effect of anabolic steroids on endurance exercise in man, but Tamaki et al. have shown a positive effect in rats.

What changes occur within the muscle itself? Blazevich and Giorgi have shown that certain changes in muscle architecture commonly associated with high-force production may be induced also by a combination of testosterone and heavy resistance training. Whilst that has little effect on muscle thickness, pennation (ability of muscle fibre to twist) and the length of muscle fibres were both increased by testosterone.

Following recent research we should then question whether:

- Further analysis of studies carried out using low doses is worthwhile; and
- More consideration should be given in studies to those anabolic steroid effects which are not directly concerned with increases in muscle strength, that is: lean body mass, psychological changes and even physical appearance. Again it must be emphasized that increases in lean body mass in runners and increased aggressiveness in American footballers and ice hockey players may be far more important to them, respectively, than improved muscle strength.

If anabolic steroid administration does produce increases in muscle strength, should this not be reflected in the progression of athletic records? Howard Payne analysed UK and world sporting records from 1950 to 1975.

The trend in all the events analysed, namely the 10 000 metres, pole vault, discus and shot shows a steady improvement year by year without a sudden upsurge in any event. Thus, anabolic steroids cannot be shown to have significantly improved performances in field events nor in the 10 000 metres, where competitors are, in some cases erroneously, assumed not to be steroid takers. A survey and review by Norton and Olds suggests that many other factors may be involved in these improvements in performance, such as improved training, selection and diet.

## Effects on Aerobic Performance

Because anabolic steroids increase haemoglobin concentration, it has been suggested that they may be able to enhance aerobic performance by improving the capacity of the blood to deliver oxygen to the exercising muscle. However, only two out of ten recent studies support this hypothesis and one actually suggests that steroids may reduce aerobic power. Tamaki et al. showed that anabolic steroids could increase exercise tolerance in rats.

## Effects on Behaviour

If, even in the most careful experiments, the positive effects of anabolic steroids are seen only in maximally exercising individuals, why is it that so many claims are made for them? One reason is possibly that steroids make them 'feel better'. Some athletes claim they feel more competitive and aggressive, others may feel they should run faster as they are on anabolic steroids. The increase in body weight and in circumference of leg and arm muscles may improve the athlete's self-image. Whether anabolic steroids enhance aggression or competitiveness is hard to assess. It is difficult to demonstrate conclusively that steroids or indeed testosterone are responsible for aggressiveness since many behaviours are probably learnt.

It is quite likely that behaviour if it is hormonally influenced is imprinted soon after birth. However, both male and female sexual behaviour are strongly influenced by androgens. Another possibility is that anabolic steroids may have a placebo effect-abusers may work or train harder because they expect anabolic steroids to work their magic! This has been investigated by Maganaris et al.. They demonstrated moderate improvements in performance in athletes who believed they were taking anabolic steroids.

## Effects on Muscle Repair

If it is agreed that anabolic steroids do increase athletic performance, albeit in strictly defined circumstances, what advantages do they confer on the taker? Obvious advantages are that the steroid taker may have stronger muscles with greater endurance, and a greater body mass with which to endure impact in sports like rugby, ice hockey or wrestling.

A further advantage conferred on the anabolic steroid taker is that their muscles and associated tissues may have greater reparative powers and so the athlete may be able to undertake more events in a short time. This observation has led to the increased use of steroids by both middle and long distance runners and marathon runners.

How does the anabolic steroid produce these effects? The original ideas that anabolic steroids simply stimulate muscle growth need to be revised following the results of the studies carried out in exercising individuals. From the results quoted previously it is possible to deduce that anabolic steroids may simply allow more intense exercise to take place thus stimulating muscle growth. Again, it could be that muscle produces an endogenous factor which stimulates further muscle growth or that exercise induces increased production of the hormones such as insulin, growth hormone and somatomedins, each of which is able to increase protein synthesis, particularly in muscle.

It is interesting that most major studies involving anabolic steroids, with the exception of that by Hervey et al., have failed to measure other hormones simultaneously. This study by Hervey et al. measured testosterone and cortisol during the treatment of athletes with methandienone. They showed that as testosterone was suppressed by methandienone treatment by the end of the experiment so plasma cortisol concentration rose. It is not clear whether this is the free, or total cortisol in the plasma, but the deduction made was that anabolic steroid effects are possibly mediated via a rise in cortisol concentration. The authors claimed that the puffy facial and thoracic features produced by anabolic steroids are similar to those occurring in Cushing's disease (CD) in which plasma cortisol is abnormally high as the result of either a pituitary or adrenocortical tumour causing adrenocortical overproduction of cortisol. There are many objections to this ingenious theory.

The symptoms of CD and anabolic steroid administration are far from similar: CD patients have a characteristic moon face, abnormal fat distribution and distended abdomen. The limb muscles are thin and wasted-producing the characteristic 'lemon on sticks' appearance of CD. More importantly, the plasma cortisol levels in CD are much greater than those quoted by the authors at the end of the study. Following Hervey's original hypothesis, other theories have suggested that anabolic steroids may block the action of cortisol and corticosterone on muscle by competing with them for their intracellular receptors. Cortisol and corticosterone inhibit muscle protein synthesis and enhance muscle protein catabolism. If this action were inhibited then muscle protein anabolism would be enhanced. Evidence for anabolic steroid binding to glucocortioid (GC) receptors has been summarized by Rockhold. Such theories of anabolic effects produced by antagonism of GC receptors must account for the observation that androgen and GC receptor numbers increase during training regimes that increase muscle mass but not during those that increase endurance.

These theories have also been analysed by Wu who concluded that in cases where individuals are insensitive to androgens because of an androgen receptor defect, supraphysiological/clinical doses of testosterone were able to reverse the muscle wasting normally associated with the condition. Anabolic steroids clearly have pharmacological effects not associated with binding to androgen cytoplasmic receptors. Whether these effects, seen only at supraphysiological/clinical doses, are mediated via cell surface receptors, glucocorticoid receptors or from displacement of testosterone and other androgens from their plasma protein binding sites remains to be established.

## THE STRANGE CASE OF CLENBUTEROL

Just before the start of the Barcelona Olympics in 1992, two British weightlifters, Andrew Saxton and Andrew Davis, tested positive for the drug clenbuterol. During the games the IOC acted swiftly to proscribe the drug. Clenbuterol is classed as a β2 -agonist; it is structurally related to salbutamol and in some EC countries (but not the UK) is similarly licensed for the treatment of asthma. However, the reason for banning the drug was associated with claims that it increased muscle mass while simultaneously reducing body fat.

β2 -Agonists can promote normal skeletal muscle growth and experiments with clenbuterol show that it can increase muscle weight in rats by 10-12 per cent after 2 weeks treatment and can reduce amino acid loss from incubated muscle. It has been shown that clenbuterol can reverse experimentally induced muscle fibre atrophy by increasing muscle protein synthesis as well as inhibiting amino acid loss. In contrast, salbutamol has no significant effect on muscle protein, though this difference may be related to the short half-life of salbutamol, since continuous infusion of salbutamol causes similar anabolic effects to clenbuterol.

Clenbuterol does not produce its anabolic effects by interacting with testosterone, growth hormone or insulin, but via β2 -receptor stimulation. Similarly the fat mobilizing action of clenbuterol is also mediated via β2 -receptors. However, the dose of clenbuterol required in animal studies to bring about an 'anabolic' effect is approximately 100 times the maximum dose that humans can tolerate.

This clenbuterol mystery seems no nearer to being solved partly because of the dual difficulties of extrapolating animal studies to man and designing ethically suitable human studies. Spann and Winter reviewed the most recent clenbuterol experiments in 1995. They analysed data from the US Department of Agriculture which demonstrated increases in muscle mass and lean body mass in steers treated with clenbuterol; a result which has also been found in rats, poultry and sheep. Human studies are much more equivocal and show that clenbuterol produces no statistically significant increase in involuntary muscle strength but that certain type II or fast-twitch muscle fibres may benefit from the drug. There is also some weak evidence that clenbuterol may improve limb muscle strength rehabilitation after an orthopaedic operation.

## THERAPEUTIC USE OF CLENBUTEROL

Clenbuterol is not licensed in the UK, but in some EC countries it is licensed for the treatment of asthma. The fact that it increases lean body mass, decreases fat and may increase muscle protein synthesis suggests that the drug may be useful in weaning anabolic steroid abusers off their drugs. Most recent evidence suggests that clenbuterol does reduce body fat and increase muscle mass, though whether this leads to a consistent increase in strength does not seem to have been demonstrated yet. The important point to be considered here is whether clenbuterol confers any athletic advantage. It is assumed that reductions in body fat and increases in lean body mass will confer advantages to most athletes. The positive 'anabolic' effects, while not yet associated with increases in strength, may be advantageous in maintaining the anabolic effects of anabolic steroids when these are withdrawn before an athletic event so as to avoid detection by doping tests. The association between clenbuterol, other β2 -agonists and gains in muscle strength in athletes warrants further investigation.

## PRECURSORS, NANDROLONE AND METABOLITES

The biosynthesis and metabolism of testosterone, and it can be seen that testosterone is produced naturally in the testis and adrenal cortex by the conversion of dehydroepiandrosterone (DHEA) to androstenedione and then to testosterone. For some years, both these substances were suggested as possible anabolic agents in the knowledge that when administered, they could be converted to testosterone in the body. Androstenedione was the major substance that Mark McGuire admitted to abusing in his quest for baseball fame in 1997-1998. Though several researchers, including the infamous East Germans, claimed that androstenedione and DHEA produced increases in serum testosterone concentration of up to 300 per cent in women and 200 per cent in men, this has not been correlated yet with any increases in muscle strength or athletic performance.

Despite this, DHEA and androstenedione were prohibited by the IOC in 1996. Brian Wallace and his colleagues showed in 1999 that compared with placebo, neither DHEA nor androstenedione was associated with a statistically significant increase in lean body mass, strength or testosterone levels. Since DHEA also disturbs the testosterone/ epitestosterone ratio, the ability to cheat with the drug seems much reduced.

This lack of androstenedione efficacy may be associated with its rapid conversion to oestrogens in peripheral tissues.

## DHT (5α-dihydrotestosterone)

This compound occurs naturally in males and females as a result of the action of the enzyme 5a-reductase on testosterone. DHT is reported to have 2-3 times the androgenic activity of testosterone and its production is necessary for normal male sexual development. As the 5a-reductase conversion is not readily reversible, the conversion of DHT to oestradiol via the 'aromatase' process is minimal, which therefore minimizes any possible feminizing effects in males, though it increases the likelihood of serious masculinizing side-effects in females. It is for this reason that the 19-nor derivative of DHT (formed by the action of 5a-reductase on nandrolone) has been suggested as a possible drug of abuse in women, as it has much less androgenic activity than DHT. Despite being promoted in the 1980s 'underground' literature as 'undetectable' doping, DHT abuse does not seem to have been identified until 1993.

Following this single case, DHT abuse was detected in 11 Chinese swimmers at the 1994 Asian Games. According to Ueki and Okana, detection is sometimes made more difficult by the simultaneous administration of 'traditional Chinese medicine', though it is unclear whether this is a deliberate attempt at masking drug abuse. DHT is still a licensed drug in some countries. It does not alter the testosterone/ epitestosterone ratio but it can be detected by examining the ratio of the urinary concentration of DHT and its 5a-metabolites to non-5a-steroids.

## Nandrolone

Nandrolone was introduced as an anabolic steroid in the 1970s. It has structural modifications that allow it to be injected intramuscularly and which also reduce the likelihood of its conversion to oestrogen by aromatase enzymes. In addition, nandrolone can be converted by the enzyme 5α-reductase to 'dihydro-19-nor-testosterone' (dihydro-nandrolone) which has even less androgenic activity and is therefore promoted as a potential 'drug of choice' for women athletes. Nandrolone is converted also to the metabolites norandrosterone and noretiocholanone by the same enzyme systems that metabolize testosterone and these components, like their respective testosterone metabolites, may be detected in urine.

The current controversy surrounding nandrolone does not only centre on the drug itself after being banned by the IOC in 1976, but on the possibility that it could be formed in the human body, by ingestion of one of its precursors, either deliberately or unintentionally. In 1997, the US Drug Enforcement Agency noticed an increase in the importation of so-called nandrolone precursors norandrostenediol and norandrostenedione into the USA. Research showed that this seemed to be coupled to advertisements on the Internet claiming that these two compounds could be converted to nandrolone in humans. In theory it should be possible to convert norandrostenedione to 19-nortestosterone (nandrolone) in humans and this has only recently been established.

As interest in nandrolone increased and even more sensitive analytical techniques appeared in the late 1990s, a new, short-acting, orally active form of nandrolone, nandrolone sulphate, was introduced. Suddenly, several high-profile nandrolone-positive test results appeared in the press involving the British Olympic Gold medallist Linford Christie, and the UK 400 m athlete Dougie Walker.

By the mid-1990s, it had been observed that the nandrolone metabolites norandosterone and noretiocholanone could be detected in the urine of previously drug-free monkeys. Also the progestogen, norethisterone, an ingredient of some oral contraceptives, was shown to increase levels of nandrolone metabolites in urine and it has also been shown that the urinary concentration of norandrosterone and noretiocholanone increases in some pregnant women. Based on this and other analytical evidence the IOC set urinary concentration limits for nandrolone metabolites at 2 ng/ml for men and 5 ng/ml for women.

Several questions arise from this controversial era of abuse testing and regulation. Since testing for nandrolone abuse either from direct administration or from precursors depends on the detection of nandrolone metabolites, are the IOC threshold levels correct? The answer to this is not clear. Nandrolone metabolites are found in urine from previously drug-free human males at a concentration below the 2 ng/ml IOC threshold.

Evidence that this is a truly endogenous production comes from the demonstration that nandrolone metabolite levels in male urine can be increased following an injection of hCG which stimulates androgen release from the testis. However, in 1999 LeBizec et al. found that while nandrolone concentrations in half of the 40 samples they tested ranged from 0.05-0.6 ng/ml, these values could be increased by a factor of 2-4 after prolonged intense exercise. Recent research by Schmitt et al. has demonstrated that exhaustive exercise does not increase the excretion of nandrolone. Could nandrolone and its metabolites be formed in humans in other ways? There was evidence in the 1980s that methosterone could be converted to a nandrolone metabolite.

Other studies have shown that pregnant women may produce increased amounts of the metabolites because of the action of hCG on the ovary. We know that hCG can stimulate production of nandrolone metabolites, but this may merely confirm that it is hCG that is being abused. Other doubts concern the claim that some vitamin and food supplements may contain trace amounts of the nandrolone precursors norandrostenedione and norandronstenediol, which are metabolized to nandrolone and then to its metabolites, thus producing a positive, super-threshold test result. To test this explanation Catlin et al. administered trace amounts of androstenedione or 19-norandrostenedione to 41 healthy men. Twenty of the 24 men receiving androstenedione yielded urine samples containing norandrosterone at a concentration above the IOC limit.

Some evidence of impurities and or norandrostenedione was found in the OTC samples. In October 2000, the IOC commissioned the Institute of Biochemistry in Cologne to investigate nutritional supplementation in sport. A total of 634 non-hormonal nutritional supplements obtained from most EU countries and from the USA were examined and analysed.

Twenty-three samples (24.5 per cent) contained precursors of nandrolone and testosterone, 64 samples (68.1 per cent) contained precursors of testosterone, while 7 samples contained nandrolone precursors only. Sample products that tested positive for anabolic steroid precursors originated from The Netherlands (25.8 per cent), Austria (22.7 per cent), the UK (18.9 per cent) and the USA (18.8 per cent). Analysis of the positive samples yielded anabolic steroid precursor concentrations of 0.01-190 μg/g. When positive-testing supplements were administered so that the total androgen intake exceeded 1 μg, the urine samples of the volunteers contained anabolic steroid levels in excess of IOC regulations. This has led to proposals for nutritional supplements to be controlled by the IOC. We can summarize that

- Nandrolone metabolites and possibly nandrolone are produced naturally in human males and females;
- Norandrosterone and norandrostenedione can be converted in humans to nandrolone metabolites
- The 2 ng cut off for nandrolone metabolites in the IOC test is fair but more studies need to be done on the effect of prolonged exercise on nandrolone secretion and the urinary concentration of nandrolone metabolites.

The questions still remain: why should exercise increase endogenous nandrolone (metabolite) production and why are there nandrolone precursors in some dietary supplements? The general side-effects of anabolic steroids. Of these side-effects some are of particular significance to athletes taking steroids, namely cardiovascular side-effects since exercise imposes a particular stress on the cardiovascular systems, and hepatic side-effects because anabolic steroids, particularly those with C-17 alkyl substituents are suspected hepatic carcinogens in the doses in which they are taken by athletes.

## Cardiovascular

Rockhold has examined nine studies on the effect of anabolic steroids on blood volume. Eight of these studies were carried out on non-athletes and produced variable results. Some studies showed increases in blood volume while others demonstrated no change. In the single study carried out in athletes a 15 per cent increase in total blood volume in athletes taking methandienone was recorded. This study did not measure haematocrit and so any effect of the steroid on erythropoiesis could not be determined.

## SALT AND WATER RETENTION

The effect of anabolic steroids on salt and water retention was discussed in relation to steroid-induced gains in body weight and muscle circumference. The increase in salt and water retention responsible for these changes has a deleterious effect on the cardiovascular system. Thus, the increased blood sodium concentration causes a rise in blood osmotic pressure. Since sodium ions cannot diffuse into cells, they remain in the extracellular fluid and blood unless excreted by the kidney, thus raising osmotic pressure and withdrawing water from the tissues. An expansion of the blood volume then occurs which imposes an increased workload on the heart. The heart increases its output and the blood pressure rises. The increased sodium concentration may also directly stimulate vasoconstriction, thus enhancing the hypertensive effect of the increased blood volume.

## HYPERTENSION

An increased incidence of potentially fatal hypertension in athletes on anabolic steroids is frequently mentioned in early reviews of anabolic steroid abuse in sport. According to Rockhold, the evidence for this is equivocal. He mentions three studies, two in athletes, one in healthy men, in which administration of either testosterone or oxandrolone for three months failed to cause an increase in blood pressure. An earlier study by Holma found a 15 per cent increase in blood volume in men taking methandienone but no increase in blood pressure. However, Kuipers et al. found mean increases in blood pressure of 12 mmHg in athletes self-administering various anabolic steroids. In a second double-blind study, using only nandrolone decanoate, no increase in blood pressure could be detected. The association between blood pressure and anabolic steroid abuse warrants further careful investigation, particularly in relation to the suggestion by Rockhold that an increased hypertensive effect might be associated with specifie types of anabolic steroid molecule.

## Ventricular function

Studies in animals on the effect of anabolic steroids on ventricular function and morphology have indicated an association between steroids and ventricular pathology which may have significance for humans particularly as the autopsy of an American footballer who was abusing anabolic steroids revealed significant cardiomyopathy. The technique of echocardiography has revolutionized non-invasive investigation of cardiac function and allows clinicians to measure accurately the dimensions of the ventricles during exercise and at rest at each stage of the cardiac cycle.

A survey of six studies of ventricular function in athletes from different disciplines abusing anabolic steroids has been conducted by Rockhold. The overall conclusion was that in intensely training athletes steroid administration induced left ventricular thickening, increases in end diastolic volume and relaxation index. Deligiannis and Mandroukas have shown that such changes occur in relation to increases in skeletal muscle mass. Nieminen et al. have reported similar cardiopathpology in four young weightlifters with cardiac hypertrophy.

Two patients additionally had symptoms of heart failure and one of these had a massive thrombosis in both ventricles. It should be noted that all the above studies were carried out in weightlifters and so may not be relevant to all athletes and it is interesting that while endurance athletes have a significantly greater life expectancy than non-athletes, this advantage is not shared by power athletes. The fact that, so far, only isolated cases of cardiomyopathy have occurred in athletes abusing steroids should serve as a warning rather than a comfort.

## EFFECTS ON BLOOD LIPIDS AND LIPOPROTEINS

Anabolic steroids have important effects on the plasma levels of triglycerides, cholesterol and lipoproteins. Lipoproteins are large molecular conglomerates of lipids and specialized proteins called apolipoproteins. Their presence in the blood is to carry water-insoluble lipids from their site of production to tissues where they are utilized or stored. Anabolic steroids have been shown to increase blood triglyceride and cholesterol levels. They decrease the blood levels of high-density lipoprotein (HDL), especially the HDL2 and HDL3 fractions, while increasing the level of low-density lipoprotein (LDL). In addition, there is a significant rise in the ratio of free cholesterol to HDL-bound cholesterol following anabolic steroid administration, though the effect is less pronounced with testosterone.

These changes appear to be induced by an action of anabolic steroids on key liver enzymes such as lipoprotein lipase and hepatic lipase associated with lipoprotein metabolism. Several studies, especially the widely quoted Framingham study in the USA, have shown that a reduction of just 10 per cent in the blood concentration of HDL could increase the chances of coronary disease by 25 per cent. A more recent study by Costill et al. has shown that in athletes taking anabolic steroids, HDL fell by 20 per cent after only 102 days of treatment, while cholesterol concentration was unchanged; while Rockhold reports even greater percentage reductions, i.e. HDL down 52 per cent, HDLb down 78 per cent. In normal males 22 per cent of cholesterol is in the form of HDL while in steroid takers only 7.8 per cent of cholesterol is found combined in this way.

There is wide agreement that anabolic steroids cause a reduction in the serum HDL cholesterol and that this phenomenon is particularly associated with the abuse of orally administered steroids. At least two recent reviews of the literature concluded that this effect of HDL is reversible, i.e. HDL levels return to normal within 3-5 weeks of cessation of steroid administration. A controlled study by Millar in which moderate doses of anabolic steroids were administered by physicians reported decreases in HDL and an increase in total cholesterol levels, which returned to normal 6-12 weeks after the end of dosage.

These reductions in HDL levels have been associated with increased incidence of cardiovascular disease in the general population. Low serum HDL is recognized as a risk factor for cardiac and cerebrovascular disease. There are several well documented cases of coronary heart disease (CHD) in apparently fit, healthy athletes aged under 40, who have been taking anabolic steroids. However, according to Lukas, only one case of an athlete dying of coronary heart disease while abusing anabolic steroids had been reported up to 1992.

It could be interpreted that low serum HDL is not a significant risk factor for steroid abusers, but it is also possible that such individuals may be fitter than the rest of the population so that any pathological changes are delayed. Street et al. in their review of anabolic steroid side-effects produced a table of individual cases of serious medical conditions associated with anabolic steroid abuse quoted in medical journals. Although, again, there was only one death due to myocardial infarction, there were several 'near misses' including five myocardial infarctions, one stroke, two cases of pulmonary embolism and one cerebral venous thrombosis. The statistics are also complicated by the different drug administration regimes used by abusers and complications arising from other risk factors such as smoking. This subject requires intensive long-term study.

## BLOOD CLOTTING

The increased risk of coronary and cerebrovascular disease in anabolic steroid abusers has prompted some physicians to consider whether there is increased risk of platelet aggregation leading to increased blood clot formation. Animal studies suggest that there is such a relationship, but so far there is only one report of an athlete taking steroids dying of a stroke, though Street et al. quote three cases of near deaths from pulmonary embolism and one venous thrombosis. However, there is an association between increased platelet aggregation and age in weightlifters taking steroids.

### Carcinomas

The association between anabolic steroid administration and tumour formation, particularly of the liver and kidney, is now firmly established. Significant changes in liver biochemistry have been found in 80 per cent of otherwise healthy athletes taking anabolic steroids but without any signs of liver disease. In 1965, a detailed case study was published linking the death of an anabolic steroid-taking athlete with hepatocellular cancer (HC). Since then 13 other athletes taking anabolic steroids have been demonstrated to have HC and all were taking 17-alkylated androgens. A second more insidious liver pathology, petiocis hepatis was associated with anabolic steroids in 1977. In this disorder hepatic tissue degenerates and is replaced by blood-filled spaces.

Anabolic steroids have also been suspected of causing death from Wilm's Tumour of the kidney in at least two adult athletes. The tumour is very rare in post-adolescent individuals. Surprisingly, in their survey of serious reported anabolic steroid side-effects, Street et al. could find only one case of prostate carcinoma. Three large case-controlled studies have found a much stronger though not unequivocal link between raised anabolic steroid levels and prostate cancer. In all three investigations, testosterone was associated significantly with an increased risk of prostate carcinoma.

## SEX-RELATED SIDE-EFFECTS

### Fertility

In the introduction it was noted that spermatogenesis in human males is under the control of gonadotrophins and testosterone. Administration of anabolic steroids caused inhibition of gonadotrophin secretion followed by inhibition of testosterone. Holma administered 15 mg of methandienone to 15 well-trained athletes for 2 months. During the administration period sperm counts fell by 73 per cent and in three individuals azoospermia was present. In those individuals with sperm present in their sample there was a 10 per cent increase in the number of immotile sperm and 30 per cent decrease in the number of motile sperm.

Thus fertility was severely reduced in males in this study, which provides confirmation of many clinical reports of the same phenomena. However, many of these effects were shown to be reversible. Though it is obviously unethical to test this, some clinical data suggest that long-term anabolic steroid-induced infertility might be permanent, though in their review of published work up to 1995, Street et al. found no evidence of long-term effects in fertility on young males given anabolic steroids to suppress excessive growth.

### Effects on Libido

The suppression of testosterone secretion in both males and females may well have effects on libido. Libido in males and females is thought to be influenced, at least in part, by testosterone. Thus, high levels of anabolic steroids in the blood suppress testosterone secretion and reduce libido. However, Yates et al. using doses of testosterone up to 500 mg per week could find no significant changes in male libido during a 14-week administration period.

### Gynaecomastia

This is a paradoxical condition occurring in athletes attempting to increase their muscle mass, as it involves the development of mammary tissue. The most common cause of this condition in anabolic steroid abusers is that the agent they are administering is converted by liver aromatase enzymes to oestradiol, which then induces development of mammary tissue. Thus athletes who abuse anabolic steroids or testosterone are at risk from developing gynaecomastia. It is widely assumed by steroid abusers that use of an anabolic steroid which cannot be aromatized to oestradiol will reduce the incidence of gynaecomastia, but there is no evidence for this. Concurrent administration of the anti-oestrogen, tamoxifen, is thought by many abusers in both the US and Britain to be an effective antidote to gynaecomastia induced by steroids. Though it is sometimes effective in reducing the pain associated with this condition, tamoxifen seems to have little effect on the size of breast tissue in steroid abusers.

## Specific Actions in Female Athletes

Considering the side-effects mentioned in the introduction, people often wonder why female athletes should take anabolic steroids. The simple answer is that women's athletics is now as competitive as men's and that, according to some reports, the effects of anabolic steroids on muscle strength and bulk in a female athlete are considerably greater than in men. This has been explained by the lower normal circulating level of testosterone in females compared with men. Thus some female athletes take anabolic steroids in the knowledge that they may produce greater muscle strength and bulk at the expense of irreversible change, such as deepening of the voice and clitoral enlargement.

In 1996, Korkia interviewed 15 female body builders who admitted to anabolic steroid abuse, nine of whom reported deepening of the voice, eight to menstrual problems and seven to clitoral enlargement. Three complained of reduction in breast size, while the other side-effects mentioned were similar to males. Side-effects such as menstrual problems are not necessarily indicative of anabolic steroid abuse as regular intense endurance exercise is known to induce amenorrhoea.

Pricilla Choi described the case of a female bodybuilder who, as a result of chronic anabolic steroid abuse, became permanently masculinized and 8 years after cessation of anabolic steroid abuse, her enlarged clitoris and her deep voice remained and she appeared to be suffering psychologically from a gender identity crisis.

### Tendon Damage

Several researchers have noted the increased incidence of

tendon damage in athletes taking anabolic steroids. A summary of the various tendon pathologies associated with anabolic steroid abuse has been provided by Laseter and Russell. These include the quadriceps and rectus femoris tendons and the triceps; the four cases all involved powerlifters. This phenomenon has been explained in at least three different ways. First, that the increase in muscle strength acquired by a course of steroids, plus training, produces a greater increase in muscle power than in tendon strength since tendons respond slowly to strength regimes and anabolic steroids have little or no effect on tendon strength.

Second, it is thought that anabolic steroids have, in common with corticosteroids the ability to inhibit the formation of collagen, an important constituent of tendons and ligaments. Third, anabolic steroids appear to induce changes in the arrangement and contractility of collagen fibrils in tendons, leading to critical alterations in physical properties known as the 'crimp angle'. The overall effect is to reduce the plasticity of the tendons. It should be pointed out that tendon ruptures also occur in athletes not abusing steroids.

Weightlifters taking anabolic steroids appear to be particularly prone to muscle and tendon injuries. This has been explained by apologists for anabolic steroid abusers as evidence of greater weights being lifted. Sports doctors say it is the biochemical effects of anabolic steroids while other say that the increased aggressiveness and competitiveness induced by anabolic steroid administration causes athletes to attempt more and greater lifts with an increasingly reckless attitude to the actual mechanics of the lifting.

## Glucose Regulation

Anabolic steroid abuse has been shown to reduce glucose tolerance and increase insulin resistance. This could lead to the induction of type II diabetes. However, in this study, the glucose tolerance was still within normal limits.

Hobbs et al. found that testosterone at 300 mg per week had little effect on glucose uptake from the plasma, while the same dose of nandrolone enhanced glucose removal from the plasma. These differences were ascribed to the ability of testosterone to undergo aromatization to an oestrogen. This may be an important consideration in relation to other side-effects of anabolic steroids. Transient decreases in immunoglobulin IgA and IgG have been reported during steroid use.

## BEHAVIOURAL EFFECTS AND ADDICTION

Since the late 1940s it has been known that anabolic steroids have important influences on behaviour, but these have usually been acknowledged to be the stimulatory effects which anabolic steroids have on libido in both males and females. There is no evidence that troops of the Nazi Waffen-SS regiments were given anabolic steroids to increase aggressiveness before battle. Studies in the 1980s have suggested that anabolic steroids have reduced the depression symptoms in a number of groups of depressed patients. Alder has shown that some women suffering from post-natal depression had abnormally low testosterone levels. It is surprising, given the frequency of anecdotal reports from athletes using steroids that they experienced euphoria, general feelings of well-being, increased confidence, self-esteem, libido and energy, that until the late 1980s little systematic research into the behavioural effects of anabolic steroids had been carried out.

A review by Kashkin and Kleber cites many documented cases of increased aggression and violent behaviour, many of them reported by the abusers themselves. The same authors also report detailed cases of mild to severe psychiatric disturbances occurring in those abusing anabolic steroids ranging from impaired judgement, insomnia and agitation to panic attacks, grandiose ideas and paranoid delusions. Pope and Katz interviewed 41 body builders and football players who had used anabolic steroids. Nine of these fulfilled the DSMIIIR criteria for mood disorder and five displayed psychotic symptoms associated with steroid use. Williamson and Young describe several cases of manic episodes in athletes taking anabolic steroids.

In a number of instances depressed steroid abusers attempting to withdraw from steroid administration became manic when treated with antidepressant drugs. Since the mid-1980s, there have been increasing reports of abusers maintaining steroid administration despite repeated attempts to stop them. There are similar reports in the literature of patients on high glucocorticoid doses being unable to stop their medication. Kashkin and Kleber also produce evidence of withdrawal symptoms in some individuals who stop taking steroids and cited several studies where steroid withdrawal had resulted in clinical depression.

In a sample of men who stopped taking steroids, 12.2 per cent were diagnosed as depressed within 3 months of abstinence. Does anabolic steroid abuse lead to an increased risk of suicide? An examination of eight cases of suicide in anabolic steroid abusers by Thiblin et al. showed that depressive symptoms arising after anabolic steroid withdrawal were associated with suicide in five cases, while in the remainder depression during anabolic steroid abuse was implicated. Anabolic steroid abuse also appears to increase the risk of being murdered, as 9 of the 34 deaths among anabolic abusers quoted by Pärssinen and Seppälä had been the victims of homicide. In Britain the suicide of a Royal Marine guardsman taking anabolic steroids was reported. These findings suggest that all anabolic steroid abusers who abstain should be carefully followed up.

There are a number of reports of steroid cravings associated with increased sympathetic nervous system activity in some abusers who attempt to refrain from anabolic steroids. There is also widespread fear, real and imaginary, of what I call 'muscle melt down', in those considering or attempting to withdraw from steroid abuse. This appears from the literature to involve feelings of loss of esteem, both social and sexual, if the well-developed torso is seen to 'melt away' after steroid withdrawal. Kashkin and Kleber consider that all the clinical evidence so far suggests the existence of a 'sex steroid hormone dependence disorder' which obeys the following established criteria for addiction:

- The hormones are used over longer periods than desired;
- Attempts are made to stop without success.
- Substantial time is spent obtaining, using or recovering from the hormones.
- Use continues despite acknowledgement of the significant psychological and toxicological problems caused by the hormones.
- Characteristic withdrawal symptoms occur.
- Hormones (or their supplements) are taken to relieve the withdrawal symptoms.

The evidence assembled by Kashkin and Kleber and Williamson and Young is substantial and convincing, but as Lukas has emphasized, the majority of athletes and body builders do not report major psychiatric symptoms, or perhaps refrain from doing so. It is interesting to note that, up to 2001, there is only one documented case of a female abuser of anabolic steroids suffering from dependency. Why does dependency occur, and only in some abusers? To answer this question Kirk Brower has summarized the theoretical biochemical and physiological and psychological factors that he thinks may influence the development of dependency. He has divided these into:

- Positive reinforcement mechanisms involving brain centres that mediate sexual function and pleasure including central opioid and dopaminergic systems, which are reinforced by
- Muscular development giving rise to psychological, social and vocational benefits. There are then in parallel:
- Negative reinforcement mechanisms-avoidance of depressive and other withdrawal symptoms which may be biologically mediated via testosterone deficiency or reduced activity of the opioid and/or dopaminergic sytems in the brain coupled with
- Psychosocially mediated mechanisms-as a psychological response to loss of muscle and loss of social/vocational rewards.

One of the major reasons proposed by steroid abusers for the use of these drugs in their sport is that it increases their aggression. A number of studies have failed to find any relationship between endogenous testosterone levels and aggression and a review of studies of aggression and hostility comparing anabolic steroid with placebo in several groups of athletes revealed both positive and equivocal results. It would be interesting to know whether increased aggression is required in the successful sportsperson and how far this differs from that found in the unsuccessful or non-athletic population. When anger scores were compared between successful and non-successful qualifiers for the 1976 US Olympic wrestling team, the highest scores occurred in those selected, suggesting that anger may be a positive feature of wrestling but not necessarily in other sports.

Pope and Katz showed that anabolic steroid abuse was associated with increased incidence of recklessness and aggressiveness. Anecdotal reports from women published in magazines and also a number of criminal cases involving evidence of male anabolic steroid abusers towards female parties prompted Choi and Pope to examine whether anabolic steroids increased the likelihood of violent behaviour of abusers towards women.

They found a significant increase in fighting behaviour, verbal aggression and violence inflicted on females by their steroid-abusing partners compared with either non-abusers or when the abusers were not taking anabolic steroids. However, Yates et al. could detect no increases in hostility in male volunteers administered with testosterone in randomized doses of 100-500 mg for 14 weeks. The same study showed there were insignificant effects of anabolic steroids on mood, libido and sexual interest. The doses here were, however, well below those normally administered by many anabolic steroid abusers.

Perhaps the most disturbing reports of all are those linking anabolic steroids with serious crime, including murder. Lubell has documented three cases of murder where anabolic steroids were cited by the defence as the causes of their clients' behaviour, and one case in Florida where the defence (unsuccessfully) entered a plea of 'not guilty by reason of insanity' for a client who committed murder while abusing anabolic steroids. The effects of anabolic steroids on behaviour and their association with psychiatric illness and criminality appear strong, but most studies reviewed here have not demonstrated clear or quantitative relationships and none has been prospective.

It is therefore impossible to know the personality or even the psychiatric profile of the person before they began abusing steroids. It is possible that body builders and even some athletes may have psychological problems, abnormal personalities or personality disorders before they begin steroid abuse. Thus body builders may suffer from body dysmorphic syndromes (feelings that their body size/shape is inadequate). Harrison Pope's research group think they can identify a 'muscle dysmorphic syndrome' in which affected individuals become 'pathologically pre-occupied with their degree of muscularity'. This new syndrome does not fit the accepted criteria in DSM IV for body dysmorphic disorder as it involves dissatisfaction with the whole body rather than a particular structure or part. It is also unclear whether some of the symptoms described are delusional, but there does seem to be some commonality with eating disorders and some types of anxiety. Athletes may also form obsessional/perfectionist desires to be the best at all costs.

John Porcerelli and Bruce Sandler have started to investigate this by attempting to construct a psychological profile of anabolic steroid users. They were particularly interested in narcissistic personality traits in anabolic steroid abusers and compared 26 steroid-abusing and 16 non-abusing weightlifters. They found significantly higher narcissism scores and lower empathy scores amongst anabolic steroid abusers, but could not detect whether these abnormalities of personality were present before abuse took place. It was unclear whether personality disorder which would meet DSM IV criteria was present among the abusers.

We also know very little about the cultural, social and

psychological influences which affect both the developing and the adult athlete and also which of these influences may lead to psychiatric disturbance and/or drug abuse. In 1992, David Begel reviewed the most recent research in sport psychiatry and concluded that the close relationship between mental and physical phenomena in sport may account for the psychiatric problems associated with poor performance. John Raglin's recent review has suggested that the psychological profile of unsuccessful athletes is not significantly different from the normal population. Among American athletes a decrease in athletic performance is termed 'slump'. It would be interesting to know what the relationship was between 'slump' and anabolic steroid taking and whether abuse of the drugs was associated with attempts to preempt it.

A detailed and highly perceptive review of the social factors leading to anabolic steroid abuse and its increased prevalence has been carried out by Anna Wroblewska. She noted the influence of cultural icons, i.e. the change in the appearance of Hollywood heroes from the simply tall and athletic to the lean, tall, wide-shouldered, muscular torso of the present day. The body dimensions of the 'Action Man' toy have changed also from tall and athletic to broad-shouldered, tall and lean-and steroidal!

Her review concludes that the relationship between anabolic steroid abuse in athletes and non-athletes is complex and is driven by numerous factors relating to athletic success and social success to self-perception of body dimensions and potential attractiveness. She has hypothesized that the lure of 'winning (be it a race or an attractive partner) is very powerful at any age and especially so in adolescence and young men'. As an aside she notes that 'research into appearance anxiety is mainly focused on women' and presumably should include both sexes.

Michael Bahrke has summarized the current evidence for anabolic steroid-induced behavioural change and psychiatric disorder. He states that because a steroid user feels more aggressive and self-reports more aggression, it does not mean that he/she is going to behave violently or develop a mental disorder. His review also emphasizes that only a a small percentage of anabolic steroid users appear to experience symptoms of mental illness. Of those that do, the majority recover without relapse when the anabolic steroids are withdrawn. It appears from this review that many methodological issues concerning this type of research need to be resolved, including sample size, dose and method of assessment.

The association between anabolic steroid abuse and all aspects of behaviour, personality and psychiatric disorder, in sport, should be the subject of continuing and further careful study.

## LONG-TERM RISKS OF ANABOLIC STEROID ABUSE

Exactly how long the Anabolic Steroid Sorcerer has cast his spell (or curse) is unknown, but if 50 years is a reasonable estimate then we should now be investigating or realizing the long-term effects of their abuse. Mortality studies are notoriously difficult to control and in the case of anabolic steroid abuse the confirmation of abuse and its intensity is difficult to verify. A study of 62 elite powerlifters in Finland emphasizes the apparent long-term effects of anabolic steroid abuse. These athletes were the prizewinners in the Finnish championships and were followed up for 12 years and compared with a control population. Premature death was 4.6 times higher in the powerlifters than in the control population. As powerlifting does not itself cause an increase in mortality, the increase in mortality in this group was ascribed to anabolic steroid abuse.

## INDIRECT CONSEQUENCES OF ANABOLIC STEROID ABUSE

Many of the surveys quoted suggest that abuse of orally active steroids is declining in favour of the injectable varieties. This may be due to better awareness of the toxicity of the oral compounds or to the supposedly lower risk of detection with injectable compounds once treatment is stopped. It is surely no coincidence that this switch appears to be associated with the appearance of HIV among steroid abusers, the first case of which was reported in the USA 18 years ago. There have been several further cases reported subsequently in body builders in the USA. The potential for the spread of HIV by this route in Great Britain has been highlighted by Perry et al. who reported high-risk behaviour, i.e. needle sharing and drug sample sharing, with all the attendant risks of cross-contamination of drug supplies and abusers' blood in their sample of body builders in Swansea.

Other related high-risk behaviour such as abuse of other more dangerous drugs, drink-driving, reckless driving behaviour and high-risk sexual activity have been catalogued in anabolic steroid abusers by Middleman and DuRant.

Another unforeseen consequence of anabolic steroid abuse by injection is tissue and organ damage caused by inexperienced and untrained injectors. There are several anecdotal cases reported to me by local GPs of 'steroid limp'. This condition is characterized by the patient who can only raise his affected leg to walk by using his abdominal adductor muscles. It is caused by damage to the sciatic nerve by injection of anabolic steroids in the but-tocks either into or close to the sciatic nerve resulting usually in permanent neuromuscular impairment.

## EDUCATIONAL AND SOCIAL ASPECTS

Though the number of positive steroid tests at Olympic events appear to be static, the high level of anabolic steroid usage by body builders and weightlifters and the disturbing level of abuse by the young in the USA and Britain shows that much remains to be done to counteract the anabolic steroid problem. The imposition of mandatory testing while possibly contributing to the decline in anabolic steroid usage in top class athletes will have little influence on the school or college abuser. In the USA mandatory testing measures have been introduced at school and college level resulting in a number of positive tests. How can the abuse be combated and how should the abuser be treated? It seems that we must first understand who is abusing and why.

Though it cannot be condoned, it is easy to understand why athletes are tempted to cheat in order to run faster or throw further, particularly with the substantial financial rewards that go with winning. It is less easy to understand why athletes will risk disqualification and gamble on their own health to achieve this.

European soccer appeared to be steroid free until the detection of anabolic steroid abuse by Dutch soccer players in 2001, including the ex-Manchester United player Jaap Stam. Perhaps it is the potential loss of all this, consequent on being tested positive, which is a disincentive. The abuse of anabolic steroids by body builders and others for cosmetic reasons is also difficult to understand, especially when they are well acquainted with the long- and short-term side-effects and have even expressed concern about them recently.

In the USA the problem has been tackled by utilizing education programmes in colleges, schools and gymnasia and encouraging medical practitioners to adopt a sympathetic attitude to steroid abusers, particularly by advising on and treating side-effects of anabolic steroids. Central to this has been a planned intervention for abusers proposed by Frankle and Leffers including psychiatric intervention, group education at gyms, schools and colleges, drug testing for competitive athletes at all levels and a problem-related counselling approach emphasizing the relationship between steroid use and side-effects.

They concluded that legal restraints on anabolic steroid supply are necessary, but more stringent legislation should be kept in the background. A similar approach has been adopted in the UK. Perry et al. have described a local project in West Glamorgan in which powerlifters in private gymnasia have been counselled, in order to prevent the spread of HIV by the sharing of contaminated drug samples and infected needles. They also advocate a sympathetic approach by GPs involving counselling, advice and support, the option of routine health checks and the admission of steroid abusers to needle-exchange schemes.

An enlightened and thoughtful local scheme for education

about, and the containment of, the anabolic steroid problem in the Durham area of North-East England has been described by Dawson. This project's aim was risk awareness and harm minimization rather than stricture. It was found that 60 per cent of participants in the local needle-exchange scheme were anabolic steroid abusers rather than heroin addicts! It was discovered that people seeking help from the scheme were in four major categories:

- Sport performance enhancers.
- Those absorbed recently into 'gym' culture.
- Occupational users, club door-men, police, prison warders.
- Cosmetic users.

This service provides direct contact between doctors and patients/abusers allowing the communication of non-judgemental advice on harm reduction, e.g. moving towards less toxic/damaging drug forms and eventually away from anabolic steroids altogether.

How successful this has been we do not know, but it may be a way forward, in particular if it invokes improved trust between physician and abuser and at last includes recognition by local and governmental authorities that there is a joint problem that we can solve together.

Have the education schemes worked? The answer appears to be a rather dejected 'no' from Yesalis and Bahrke in their review of adolescent anabolic steroid abuse. They conclude emphatically that 'scare tactics' have no role in persuading youth not to abuse steroids. When 3-12 per cent of adolescent US males continue to abuse steroids any complacency is misplaced. They feel targeting social influences may be more beneficial. Some support for this comes from the report by Goldberg et al. on the effectiveness of the 'Adolescents training and learning to avoid steroids programme' in the USA.

Though at the end of the first year of the programme anabolic steroid abuse had not fallen significantly in the 3207 adolescent athletes surveyed, there were reductions in the abuse of alcohol, amphetamines and use of supplements, indicating that progress could be made here using sex-specific, team-centred education. The continuing mean prevalence of anabolic steroid abuse of 1.1 per cent in the US adolescent athletic population indicates that there is much still to be done. According to the survey by Faigenbaum et al. 54 per cent of US high school students who abused anabolic steroids knew they were harmful.

With the age of first use being as low as 12-13 years in some studies it is obvious that these educational programmes must start at a very early age. Many longitudinal studies are now active in the USA to study trends in drug abuse, including the MTF study, the Youth Risk and Behaviour Surveillance System (YRBSS) and the National Household Survey on Drug Abuse (NHSDA), and their techniques and reports have been analysed by Yesalis et al.. It is hoped that the information they gather may be used to plan future strategies.

Anabolic steroids were reclassified as controlled drugs in Great Britain in 1994, but this may not be the answer to the UK problem. A sensible compromise might be the compulsory licensing of all local authority leisure centres and private gymnasia.

The worrying trend of increasing anabolic steroid abuse in schools and colleges in the USA has been noted, but until the 1990s has been unrecognized in Great Britain. The survey in Scotland by Williamson emphasized that such complacency was misplaced as 56 per cent of those admitting to steroid abuse began doing so when 17 or younger. It was also important that this survey identified a significant number (50 per cent) who were regular rugby union players, athletes who were previously 'not usually recognized' as steroid abusers. The 1998 survey of secondary age school children in Sefton, Merseyside, quoted by Dawson, revealed 6.4 per cent of boys and 1.3 per cent of girls had been offered anabolic steroids. More studies in Great Britain need to be carried out and an immediate intensive education programme centred on schools and colleges should be instigated.

Perhaps also, exercise scientists should be prepared to take the lead and adopt a more high-profile role in the fight against drug abuse in sport as suggested by Kuipers. Doctors and members of the paramedical professions are also sometimes placed in an invidious position: knowing that a patient is a sports cheat and yet bound to do their utmost to care for them and maintain confidentiality.

Are we wasting our time? Athletes are getting bigger, taller, heavier and so is the general adult population world-wide according to Kevin Norton and Tim Olds. Increasingly, athletes are being selected for size, bigness/ tallness equals success and this is mirrored in society as a whole. They state that in some sports where small stature is important, this is reducing the pool of talent available.

The next trend they suggest is genetic manipulation by direct or eugenic means. Is this the end of steroids? Will the Sorcerer return?

## Chapter 6

# Glycoprotein Hormones and Sport

### HUMAN GROWTH HORMONE

Human growth hormone (hGH) is one of the major hormones influencing growth and development in humans. Such is the complexity of human growth, a period extending from birth to the age of 20 years, that a very large number of hormones influence it, producing many complex interactions. Besides hGH, the hormones, testosterone, oestradiol, cortisol, thyroxine and insulin have important roles at different stages of growth and development. The exact role of hGH is difficult to evaluate exactly, because of the many different developmental and metabolic processes which hGH can influence.

### RELEASE OF HUMAN GROWTH HORMONE

hGH secretion is episodic, the highest levels (0.5-3.0 mg/1) occurring 60-90 minutes after the onset of sleep. hGH is metabolized in the liver; the plasma half-life is only 12-45 minutes. The physiological regulation of hGH release is complex. Systemic factors stimulating hGH secretion include hypoglycaemia, a rise in blood amino acid concentration, stress and exercise, while conversely hGH secretion is inhibited by hyperglycaemia. Both endurance exercise and resistance training have been shown to cause an increase in hGH secretion in female athletes.

The anterior pituitary, a small endocrine gland at the base of, but not part of, the brain, contains somatotroph cells which secrete growth hormone. Release of hGH is under the control of two hypothalamic hormones: somatostatin, which inhibits secretion, and somatocrinin, which stimulates its secretion. Oestradiol also stimulates hGH secretion while testosterone has very little effect. Various brain neurotransmitter systems also influence hGH secretion.

This is thought to occur via a controlling influence on the hypothalamic production of somatostatin and somatocrinin, but direct effects on the somatotroph cells cannot be ruled out. Drugs such as clonidine that stimulate α2- adrenergic receptors cause increases in hGH secretion, while drugs that stimulate β2 -receptors such as salbutamol decrease hGH secretion. The factors influencing hGH secretion have been reviewed in detail by Macintyre and Muller.

## HUMAN GROWTH HORMONE ACTION

The most obvious action of hGH is that it stimulates somatic growth in pre-adolescents, but it also has metabolic effects. The importance of these metabolic actions in homeostatic regulation of fuel usage and storage is unclear as is the overall role of hGH in the adult.

Receptors for hGH are present on the surface of every cell in the body the actions of hGH is further complicated by the involvement of the plasma growth factors or somatomedins in the action of hGH. hGH stimulates the release mainly from the liver of two hormonal polypeptides, somatomedin C (or insulin-like growth factor I) and somatomedin A (insulin-like growth factor II), and a full account of this is provided by Macintyre and Kicman and Cowan.

Somatomedin C will be known as IGF-I and somatomedin A (insulin-like growth factor II) as IGF-II. IGF-I is the most important of these IGFs but there is still doubt whether many, if any, of the important metabolic effects of hGH are mediated via IGFs.

In addition, the liver produces three binding proteins with affinity for insulin-like growth factors. These are called of which IGFBP-3 seems to be the most important. IGFs are carried in the plasma in two different forms: as ternary complexes and simpler low-molecular-weight complexes. The ternary complexes which contain the IGF in combination with IGFB-3 and a protein called ALS (acid-labile subunit) render the IGF biologically inactive, unable to enter tissue spaces and resistant to metabolism. The simple complexes, however, allow the IGFs to enter tissue spaces from the blood capillaries. Very little IGF remains free in the blood.

### Effects on Muscle

hGH seems to have some effects on muscle growth but the effect of IGF-I is greater. This action appears similar to that of insulin in that it promotes amino acid uptake and stimulates protein synthesis resulting, in children, in an increase in the length and diameter of muscle fibres, while only the latter growth occurs in adults. This stimulation of muscle protein synthesis and growth is qualitatively different to that induced by work, since insulin is required for hGH-stimulated muscle growth but not for that induced by work. However, the action of insulin is more likely to be an anti-catabolic effect on muscle protein rather than a direct stimulatory effect on muscle protein synthesis.

### Effects on Bone

hGH stimulates directly and via the IGFs the elongation of bone in pre-adolescents. This is achieved by a stimulation of cartilage proliferation in the epiphyseal plates situated at each end of each long bone. Cartilage cells possess receptors for hGH and IGFs.

### Effects on Metabolism

The actions of hGH on metabolism are complex at both the cellular and organ level and appear to be biphasic. In the first or acute phase, which seems to involve the action of hGH alone, amino acid uptake into muscle (via mobilization of muscle membrane amino acid transporters) and liver is stimulated, and there is increased glucose uptake into muscle and adipose tissue together with reduced fat metabolism. During the second, chronic phase, mediated by the IGFs, there is increased lipolysis (triglyceride breakdown) in adipose tissue resulting in a rise in the plasma concentration of fatty acids and increased fatty acid utilization, thus sparing glucose.

### Effects on Adipose Tissue

Treatment of GH-deficient adults has shown that GH can increase lean body mass by several kilograms and decrease fat mass, especially visceral fat, by an equivalent amount. Whether the same effect would be achieved in someone with normal GH secretion is unknown. Treatment with hGH causes a rise in blood free fatty acid levels or rise in the blood glucose level and a reduction in the triglyceride content of adipose tissue which contributes to a decrease in adipose tissue mass and an increase in fat-free weight.

### Effects of Exercise on hGH

It is worth considering the hGH response to exercise in more detail. Within 20 minutes of beginning exercise to 75-90 per cent VO2max, hGH levels rise. The intensity of the response depends on age, level of fitness and body composition. The type of exercise undertaken also produces varying hGH responses. Intense exercise produces earlier hGH secretion, endurance exercise produces hGH peaks in mid-term, while intermittent intense exercise is claimed to result in the highest hGH levels.

## ADMINISTRATION AND SUPPLY OF HGH

hGH is a peptide and must be injected. The same problems of possible contamination of samples and infection of needles apply as with injection of anabolic steroids. Human GH is now produced synthetically, as hGH from human sources has been withdrawn because of possible contamination with the prion agent that is thought to spread the degenerative brain disorder, Creutzfeld-Jacob disease (CJD).

Initially, synthetic, injected hGH was associated with the stimulation in the recipient of hGH antibodies. This problem has been solved by increased purification procedures. Therapeutically, hGH administration is usually recommended as either three single injections, intramuscularly (i.m.) or subcutaneously (s.c.), or daily s.c. injections in the evening. The supply of hGH is controlled by law in the UK under the Medicines Act 1968. In the USA, hGH is regulated by the Food Drug and Cosmetic Act but Congressional hearings have taken place with a view to making it a schedule II controlled substance. One of the major limitations on hGH supply is its price. It was claimed in the 1990s that abusers in the US had to spend $30 000 per year to obtain worthwhile effects. There is also some evidence that much of the hGH reaching the abuser is either counterfeit, adulterated, of animal origin or some other product.

Thus, abusers are being sold bovine hGH stolen from farms (useless in humans), other peptide hormones such as human chorionic gonadotrophin (hCG), which actually stimulates testosterone production, or even anabolic steroids themselves. Many hGH supplies are known to be illicitly obtained by theft from pharmaceutical company production lines and from retail pharmacies.

According to Macintyre a number of artificial stimuli have been used to increase hGH secretion. The ones used most frequently in clinical situations are clonidine, arginine and insulin-induced hypoglycaemia, but abusers are also known to administer gamma(ã)-hydoxybutyrate (GHB), a drug which is used as an anaesthetic in some parts of Europe but which is unlicensed in the UK.

Attempts to counteract the embargo on hGH and the increasingly pro-hibitive price have included administering drugs which stimulate hGH release such as clonidine, propranolol and bromocriptine. More legitimate means include the ingestion of the amino acids arginine, ornithine, lysine and tryptophan. Arginine is the most potent of a number of amino acids which stimulate hGH secretion. As it is a normal constituent of protein and of a balanced diet its 'abuse' would be difficult if not impossible to detect.

Some dietary products for athletes claim to be rich in arginine so as to promote hGH secretion. The long-term effectiveness of arginine and other amino acids in promoting or maintaining increases in hGH levels remains to be investigated, along with the claims made for α-hydroxybutyrate.

## Growth Hormone Disorders

Inadequate secretion of hGH is one of the causes of the condition known as dwarfism. This disorder is usually recognized in childhood when the rate of growth is below the 90 per cent percentile for that child's age, race and sex. Further tests involve 'challenges' to the pituitary in the form of arginine, clonidine or insulin. If these fail to evoke adequate hGH secretion then a diagnosis of dwarfism, due to inadequate hGH, can be made. The treatment is regular administration of synthetic hGH until the end of puberty. Treatment after adolescence is ineffective in stimulating growth in stature because by this time the epiphyseal plates in the long bones have fused, terminating any further bone growth. Overproduction of hGH as a result of a tumour may occur in puberty and adolescence when it gives rise to gigantism; the individual is well above average adult height for their age, sex and race, and the limbs and internal organs are also enlarged.

In late adulthood, a tumour of the anterior pituitary causing increased hGH secretion causes the condition known as acromegaly. The affected individual does not grow any taller because the epiphyses have fused, but their internal organs enlarge (especially the heart), the fingers grow and the skin thickens. Metabolic disorders occur which often precipitate type II diabetes mellitus.

In the past 10 years, a deficiency in hGH secretion in adulthood has been recognized in elderly people, some of whom have responded favourably to hGH therapy. The investigations of this syndrome while providing interesting data on the effects of hGH have not indicated a universal benefit for the elderly of hGH treatment.

## Therapeutic Use of hGH

hGH is used to treat pituitary dwarfism when it must be administered to the affected individual before the end of puberty. The administration must be carefully monitored to prevent diabetes and/or hyperplasia of the skin. Synthetic growth hormone is now used instead of hGH obtained from human autopsies.

It has also been suggested by a number of geriatricians that hGH might be used to reverse some of the bodily changes occurring in old age. Normal ageing is associated with a reduction in lean body mass, an increase in fat mass and a reduction in skin thickness. Trials of hGH treatment in the elderly have shown that the hormone is able to reverse these changes but a recent review of world-wide clinical trials of hGH in the elderly was not favourable. A possible role for the hormone in patients with severe burns and even AIDS is also under investigation.

## THE ABUSE OF HGH IN SPORT

There appear to be four major abuses of hGH in sport: (1) to increase muscle mass and strength, (2) to increase lean body mass, (3) to improve the 'appearance of musculature', and (4) to increase final adult height. Scientific evidence from controlled trials that hGH increases muscle strength is controversial. There is some evidence to support the claim that hGH administration may increase lean body mass. Lombardo et al. describe experiments where hGH administration has caused significant reductions in 'fat weight', and increases in fat-free weight compared with placebo.

As early as 1988, Cowart reviewed anecdotal reports by body builders of increases in strength following hGH administration. There are also several positive findings of increased muscle growth, strength and protein synthesis in hGH deficient adults treated with human growth hormone. When Taaffe examined the effects of growth hormone treatment on muscle strength and lean body mass in elderly men they found no increases in strength but an increase in lean body mass and a decrease in fat mass. Similarly when Yarasheski et al. examined resistance training schedules before and during hGH administration in elderly men they found hGH did not further enhance muscle strength improvements induced by exercise regimes. In younger adult men there is a similar picture. Sixteen healthy men, 21-34 years, who had not previously trained were given hGH (0.56 IU/kg per week) or placebo during 12 weeks of heavy resistance training.

At the end of the study, lean body mass and total body water increased in the hGH group compared with placebo, but there was no difference in muscle strength or limb circumference. Negative results have also been obtained with seven weightlifters who were given hGH at 0.56 IU/kg per week during a 14-day heavy session. Muscle protein synthesis did not increase and there was no change in whole body protein breakdown. When slightly higher doses (0.63 IU/kg per week) were administered to 22 male power athletes aged 20-28 for 6 weeks no increases in biceps or quadriceps maximal strength occurred in the hGH group compared with placebo.

What conclusions can we draw from the above evidence, which conflicts with positive anecdotal reports and the continuing popularity of hGH abuse suggested by surveys and from the infamous confiscation of hGH in the 1998 Tour de France?

By 1992, Kicman and Cowan had stated that several 'underground' advocates of hGH were commenting adversely on its usefulness and yet the abuse continues. Ehrnborg et al reviewed the experiments previously described and concluded that possibly the studies are 'too short and included too few subjects'. As with early studies on anabolic steroids the doses used may have been too low and some of the hGH abusers may also have been concurrently abusing anabolic steroids. Another conclusion advanced by Wirth and Gieck is that the experiments did use suitable subjects but that hGH is simply not a suitable ergogenic aid for weightlifters and similar athletes. It may therefore be beneficial to other athletes via mechanisms or processes not yet investigated.

Yarasheski et al. also concluded that increases in lean body mass can occur without increases in strength if it is non-contractile protein that is produced. A further complication has been advanced by William Kraemer. He is quoted by Schnirring as stating that athletes may well be combining low doses of hGH with low doses of anabolic steroids and gaining an additive effect.

It is claimed that hGH administration because of the above effects improves the appearance of the bodybuilder making his/her muscles more salient or 'sculpted' and improving their photogenicity. There is no way this effect can be measured directly or objectively but it appears to be a logical development associated with loss of fat tissue. This may be the most important effect that some abusers are seeking. Its basis needs further research, particularly in relation to psychiatric and personality factors described for anabolic steroids.

The desire to produce tall offspring for cosmetic reasons, 'so that their athletic potential is increased' where height is an advantage or so that they can qualify for a vocation where there is a minimum height limit has prompted hGH abuse amongst children in the USA. Despite the ethical problems that it presents in relation to sport, childen may later resent their tallness, particularly it later they fail to qualify as professional sportspersons for other reasons. Also, it is difficult to gauge exactly how much hGH should be given so as not to produce an overly tall individual. Other potential problems of child treatment relate to side-effects. An apparent relentless drive for 'bigness' and 'tallness' in sport and society by selective and drug-induced.

## SIDE-EFFECTS ASSOCIATED WITH HGH ABUSE IN SPORT

The potential risks of hGH therapy in children have been mentioned together with the close monitoring required in paediatric patients. In the UK, the recommended standard replacement dose of hGH is about 0.6 IU/kg body weight per week. It is widely assumed that athletes who abuse the drug are taking 10 times this dose. Major side-effects include skeletal changes, enlargement of the fingers and toes, growth of the orbit and lengthening of the jaw. The internal organs enlarge and the cardiomegaly which is produced is often one of the causes of death associated with hGH abuse. Although the skeletal muscles increase in size, there are often complaints of muscle weakness. Biochemical changes include impaired glucose regulation hyperlipidaemia and insulin resistance. At least one report, however, has found that clinical doses of hGH did not produce diabetic symptoms in children with short stature. These changes described above contribute to the prevalence of diabetes in hGH abusers. Arthritis and impotence often occur after chronic hGH abuse.

A weird consequence of the increased protein synthesis during hGH abuse is changes to the skin. This includes thickening and coarsening-the so-called 'elephant epidermis' which has been known to make the skin almost impenetrable by standard gauge syringe needles. Other skin effects include activation of naevocytes and an increase in dermal viscosity. This combination of side-effects, particularly the cardiomegaly, hyperlipidaemia and hyperglycaemia, almost certainly contributes to the shortened life span seen in those suffering from overproduction of hGH. The effect of hGH on blood lipids seems equivocal: whereas long periods of abuse may cause elevation of blood lipids, abuse for up to 6 weeks may decrease plasma cholesterol and apolipoproteins.

There are few scientific studies available on the prevalence of hGH abuse in sport. Macintyre has identified American football players and bodybuilders as the most likely abusers based on laboratory reports from accredited testing agencies. Significantly, the UK investigation into drug abuse by athletes in South Wales by Perry et al. revealed no hGH abuse. By 1997, Korkia and Stimson reported that 2.7 per cent of the anabolic steroid abusers in their UK survey were also abusing hGH, while Evans also found concordant abuse of anabolic steroids and hGH in 12.7 percent of abusers in his gymnasia survey. Presumably the co-abuse here was for the reasons cited previously; that is, possibly to reduce hyperlipidaemia side effects of anabolic steroids and for a co-operative effect on muscle strength whilst preventing the 'expected' loss of muscle strength when anabolic steroids are withdrawn.

The reasons for hGH abuse appear to be based on some false premises that it is as effective as anabolic steroids, with fewer side-effects and is less easily detected. Abusers believe hGH may protect the athlete who has abused anabolic steroids and who wishes to stop 'muscle meltdown', when anabolic steroids are withdrawn.

If abuse is difficult to identify in adults, this is not the case in adolescents. Five per cent in a recent survey admitted using hGH and 24.5 per cent claimed to know of someone who was abusing it. Fifty per cent of the abusers could not name one side-effect of hGH. Those who abused hGH were most likely to be involved in wrestling or American football and to have obtained their information about hGH from another person such as a coach. There was also some evidence of co-abuse of anabolic steroids and hGH in the same adolescent sample.

## Detection of hGH Abuse

hGH abuse in detail but some consideration of it is important because of the widespread belief that it remains undetectable. Ben Johnson, for example, only confessed to abusing hGH after he had been banned for doping with anabolic steroids! Cheating with hGH is based on the observations that administered hGH is indistinguishable from endogenous hGH and that the plasma half-life of hGH is only 15-28 minutes and less than 0.01 per cent of hGH is excreted in urine. Despite this there is a good correlation between plasma and urinary hGH concentrations which might enable recent hGH abuse to be detected during random urine sampling.

Lack of a suitable test almost certainly led to the 1996 Atlanta Olympics being labelled the 'Growth Hormone Games' by Charles Yesalis, quoted in an article by Schnirring. Advances in the detection of illicit hGH administration have been made since the last edition of this book and are reviewed in detail by Bidlingmaier et al. and Sonksen.

One method relies on immunological differences between endogenous and recombinant (biosynthetic) hGH and their detection by radioimmunoassay (RIA). However, the test will not distinguish hGH which has been injected after extraction from human cadavers or hGH released by the action of drugs that stimulate hGH release. A separate assay detects increases in plasma factors or constituents known to be influenced by hGH secretion or injection. Both these tests, unfortunately, require blood samples, which has legal and religious implications in many countries.

The two plasma factors deemed most suitable are IGF-I and IGCBP-3 and possibly also the so-called acid labile subunit (ALS) described recently by Boisclair et al.. It should be obvious that extreme care must be taken before a cheat-proof hGH/IGF test is inaugurated.

Recent research shows that hGH and IGF-1 plasma levels can be elevated following a resistance training programme. After the Sydney Olympics, the Italian evening newspaper Carriere della Sera claimed that five of their country's Gold medallists had abnormally high hGH levels before the Olympic competition. Later, when one of the female Olympic cycling champions was tested under normal and stressed conditions, it was found that stress caused a significant increase in her hGH to 1.5 times the normal level, while IGF-1 remained normal.

In 1993, the possible development of orally active hGH-releasing peptides with similar actions to somatocrinin was described. If these compounds are developed, manufactured, and marketed, they will further complicate the picture. Future alternatives to hGH may well be IGFs themselves. These are not yet available commercially, but being much smaller and simpler molecules than hGH, their synthesis by 'designer' chemists is possibly more feasible. They could be used to circumvent hGH/IGF-I/IGFBP-3 tests, or by themselves. Much will depend on how accurately clinical biochemists can distinguish the many metabolic effects of hGH from those of IGF-I alone.

## Social Factors Associated with hGH

The hGH 'problem' appeared to be mainly confined to the USA in the early 1990s, but this may be because this is the major source of information on hGH abuse in athletes. The prevalence of hGH abuse in the young (5 per cent in the survey of Rickert et al., 1992) suggests that hGH abuse is taking a hold in a small group of obsessed athletes. It is also prevalent in the UK, mainly amongst co-abusers of anabolic steroids. Educational programmes similar to those advocated for steroids. However, according to Cowart much pressure on physicians to prescribe hGH comes from parents, who will also need educating. In the USA there have already been Congressional inquiries into the law relating to hGH and a number of state legislatures such as Texas have enacted laws classifying hGH as a controlled drug.

## ADRENOCORTICOTROPHIC HORMONE (ACTH)

ACTH is produced and secreted by the corticotroph cells of the anterior pituitary. It is a polypeptide consisting of 39 amino acids, of which only the 24 N-terminal amino acids are necessary for its biological activity. ACTH stimulates the reticularis and fasciculata cells of the adrenal cortex to synthesize and secrete corticosteroids such as cortisol and corticosterone. ACTH itself is never used for treatment or abuse; instead a synthetic derivative, the peptide tetracosactrin consisting of the first 24 N-terminal amino acids of ACTH, is administered by injection. Tetracosactrin administration stimulates a rise in blood cortisol and corticosterone concentration within 2 hours.

### Abuse of ACTH

ACTH abuse is limited to short-term boosting of plasma cortisol and corticosterone in an attempt to reduce lethargy and produce 'positive' effects on mood during training and competition. It is for this reason that it is banned by the IOC along with corticosteroids. ACTH and corticosteroids are unsuitable for chronic use because they decrease muscle protein synthesis, leading to skeletal muscle wasting.

### Detection of ACTH

Tetracosactrin abuse and endogenous ACTH are difficult to detect in urine samples. In the blood a rise in ACTH levels and therefore of corticosteroids occurs naturally during exercise. Kicman and Cowan investigated blood analysis for tetracosactrin, which should enable abuse to be detected.

## INSULIN AND ITS USE IN SPORT

An innocent enquiry by a Russian medical official at the Nagano Winter Olympics in 1998 led to the investigation of insulin by sports authorities and its subsequent prohibition in non-diabetic athletes by the IOC. There are no published, scientific/clinical studies on the effects of insulin on athletic performance and so much of the rationale to explain the 'street' knowledge that insulin is ergogenic in athletics is theoretical. Insulin has powerful effects on carbohydrate, fat and protein biochemistry and simultaneously has a co-operative effect on these processes with other hormones particularly hGH and IGF-I. Insulin enhances glucose uptake into muscle and aids the formation and storage of muscle glycogen.

It inhibits glucose output from the liver; so encouraging liver glycogen storage. In adipose tissue, insulin encourages triglyceride formation and thus the formation of fat. The action of insulin on muscle and muscle protein is more complex. There has always been weak evidence that insulin increases muscle protein synthesis, but it now seems that in normal physiology, hGH and IGF-I are more important than insulin in stimulating this process. Insulin's role now seems to be inhibition of protein catabolism, an action it may share with supraphysiological doses of anabolic steroids. So what is the basis for the 'underground' enthusiasm for insulin? This can be summarized briefly as follows:

- Increasing muscle glycogen stores.
- Enhancing muscle glycogen storage during training schedules to increase stamina.
- As a co-operative muscle-building stimulant with hGH.

In example 3, insulin would enhance the effects of hGH while the latter would oppose the insulin-stimulated deposition of triglycerides in adipose tissue. A full account of the physiology of this new phase of doping is provided by Sonksen.

## HUMAN CHORIONIC GONADOTROPHIN (HCG)

Human chorionic gonadotrophin (hCG) is produced by placental trophoblast cells during pregnancy and also by a number of different types of tumour cell. Its major physiological role is stimulation of the corpus luteum in pregnant females to maintain synthesis and secretion of the hormone progesterone during pregnancy. However, when injected into males, hCG also stimulates the Leydig cells of the testis to produce testosterone and epitestosterone, and so it can mimic the natural stimulation of testicular hormone produced by luteinizing hormone (LH). Administration of hCG stimulates secretion of testosterone and epitestosterone in a 'natural' ratio, allowing the testosterone/epitestosterone test to be circumvented.

The Leydig cells of the testis possess receptors which when stimulated by LH or hCG bring about activation of testosterone synthesis. This increase in synthesis is rapid, a 50 per cent increase in plasma testosterone concentration has been measured 2 hours after i.m. injection of 6000 IU of hCG. Injection of hCG also stimulates production of nandrolone (19-nortestosterone) metabolites and this may indicate that it can stimulate production of endogenous nandrolone.

### Therapeutic Use

hCG is used to stimulate ovulation in conjunction with follicle stimulating hormone (FSH) in infertile women. Occasionally, hCG is used to stimulate testicular hormone production when puberty is delayed.

### hCG Abuse in Sport

The increasingly successful identification of anabolic steroid abusers by various IOC approved tests has led abusers to switch to testosterone abuse, which itself may be detected by measurement of the testosterone:epitestosterone ratio. hCG abuse has become popular because it stimulates the secretion from the testes of both testosterone and epitestosterone, resulting in a urinary excretion ratio of less than 6:1, below the limit set by the IOC.

This led to the banning of hCG by the IOC in 1987. A standard doping regime for hCG has been described in which the abuser first injects testosterone. Apart from any gains in strength or competitiveness the testosterone causes inhibition of LH secretion from the pituitary.

When testosterone is withdrawn before competition the athlete would be at a disadvantage with lower than normal plasma testosterone levels. However, administration of hCG stimulates testicular testosterone secretion and also that of epitestosterone, so that apparent compliance with IOC regulations occurs. In a small, elegant experiment, Kicman et al. reproduced this situation in three normal men and showed that hCG can stimulate the testosterone substitution claimed by abusers and retain the testosterone/epitestosterone ratio within the IOC limits. In all three cases, the hCG could be detected in the urine by radioimmunoassay as long as plasma testosterone levels were raised.

Brower has described three separate regimes to restore endogenous testosterone secretion to normal following its suppression by administration of testosterone or anabolic steroids. He has recorded descriptions of hCG at 50 IU/kg producing a doubling of endogenous testosterone secretion within 3-4 days of administration.

Despite the availability of a highly specific radioimmunoassay for hCG, it does not reproduce the discriminating power of GC-MS and so it is as yet unacceptable to the IOC. However, the incidence of gynaecomastia may be greater as hCG also stimulates oestradiol production by the Leydig cells. The increase of oestradiol may be linked to nandrolone metabolite production in the process of aromatization.

## Prevalence of hCG Abuse

Though hCG abuse is mentioned in the survey by Yesalis and Bahrke, it is not quantified. In two UK surveys the prevalence of hCG abuse was 22.7 per cent and 49 per cent. In an earlier UK survey in the same area as Evans, Perry et al. did not record any hCG abuse, suggesting that in the UK its abuse has occurred or been detected only in the past 5-6 years.

## LUTEINIZING HORMONE (LH) AND ITS USE IN SPORT

Luteinizing hormone (LH) is produced by the gonadotroph cells of the anterior pituitary in both males and females. In males LH stimulates testicular sperm production and the synthesis and secretion of testosterone, while in females it stimulates ovulation and the production of progesterone. There are structural similarities between LH and hCG and a detailed comparison is made by Kicman and Cowan. LH secretion is subject to negative feedback control by testosterone, i.e. as plasma testosterone levels rise, so LH secretion is reduced.

In the previous edition of this book, LH was cited as a potential drug of abuse because its stimulation of testosterone production by the testis also produces epitestosterone such that the normal testosterone to epitestosterone ratio is maintained in plasma and urine. Its abuse is limited by its scarcity

# Chapter 7

# Drug Treatment in Sports Injuries

All sports have developed from the natural capabilities of the human mind and body and so, when partaken at modest level, few sports involve great risk of physical injury. This situation changes dramatically when sporting pursuits are undertaken at higher competitive levels. As it becomes necessary to push the body further, in an effort to achieve greater performance, a point may well be reached where the stresses and strains exerted on the structural framework of the body may exceed that which the body is capable of withstanding, resulting in connective tissues being torn or joints being dislocated.

Many sports carry their own peculiar additional risks of injury to the body; the boxer may suffer repeated blows to the face causing extensive bruising and laceration and the footballer may receive kicks to the legs resulting in bruising or even bone fracture.

Any traumatic injury to a competitor will result in a reduced level of performance capability and may require the abstention from sport for a period of recuperation. As well as the pain and personal discomfort associated with injury the individual's performance is likely to deteriorate during a period of inactivity. Muscle bulk may be lost and an extended training period will inevitably be required to regain peak fitness. In a sport where a career may be of limited duration and where there is a short season of competition the result of even minor trauma may be devastating. To the keen amateur, years of training may be wasted by an inability to participate competitively in a once in a lifetime event. To the top international professional a day on the bench may represent the loss of vast sums of money to the individual or club.

Whatever the cause or nature of the injury one of its inevitable features will be the occurrence of an inflammatory reaction at the damaged site. If we are to appreciate the potential to treat sports injuries we must have some understanding of the inflammatory response.

## THE INFLAMMATORY RESPONSE

The term inflammation is derived from the Latin inflammare which means to set on fire. It is a term widely employed to describe the pathological process that occurs at the site of tissue damage. A precise definition of the condition is difficult as its nature can vary quite significantly. If we accept that it is a process which is aimed at maintaining the integrity of the tissues and that the bloodstream carries a huge range of cells and chemicals which have a role in the protection of the body, then it is feasible to construct a useful, descriptive definition.

Inflammation is a process that enables the body's defensive and regenerative resources to be channelled into tissues which have suffered damage or are contaminated with abnormal material (such as invading micro-organisms). It is a process which aims to limit the damaging effects of any contaminating material, to cleanse and remove any foreign particles and damaged tissue debris, and allow healing processes to restore the tissues to some kind of normality. Inflammation is a process which is fundamentally important for survival.

Inflammation is a phenomenon that was well known to ancient civilizations. Examples of inflammatory conditions can be identified in early writings of Chinese, Egyptian, Greek and Roman origin. Hieroglyphs that can be translated as inflammation can be identified in an Egyptian manuscript, which is about 4000 years old. The classical description of inflammation was undoubtedly given by Celsus in the first century AD. In his De re medicinia he states that 'the signs of inflammation are four, redness and swelling with heat and pain'. To these four signs was added a fifth, loss of function, by Virchow, the founder of modern cellular pathology. Loss of function is a consequence of the swelling and pain associated with inflammation and is clearly an indication that affected tissues require rest for rapid rehabilitation.

Prior to the 20th century the principal tool employed to study the processes of inflammation was the microscope. Defence mechanisms typical of those seen in mammals were found in many simple organisms and it was maintained that the primary movement of the inflammatory reaction was the direction of protoplasm to digest any noxious agent. This activity can be seen in many different phyla of the animal kingdom. In protozoans, phagocytic (engulfing) activity is exerted by the organisms as a whole, but in more complex animals this function is attributed to specialized cells. The phagocytic cells of multicellular organisms are able to move to the site of the noxious agent by amoeboid movement (a directional, flowing movement of the cytoplasm).

This movement is greatly enhanced in, but not restricted to, those organisms having a vascular system for transport of these cells to the affected area. The ability to ingest and destroy foreign, non-self material such as bacteria and to remove damaged tissue debris is vitally important. Nineteenth century physiologists recognized the importance of the circulation and proposed that it was the vascular system itself which was responsible for inflammation.

Undoubtedly the vascular system is of fundamental importance in the inflammatory process of mammals, but it is well to remember that defensive reactions can occur in simple organisms which do not possess a vascular system. The reaction of such organisms to noxious stimuli will not, however, be accompanied by all the classic signs of inflammation. Without a vascular system there can be no redness or heat, and indeed with the exception of mammals and birds, which are warm blooded, inflammation of the tissues in animal species will not be accompanied by heat at the affected site.

Inflammation is a dynamic process, and this process may,

on occasions, be capable of causing more harm to the organism than the initiating noxious stimulus itself. The necrotic lesions produced on dogs at the feeding site of a tick, for example, are brought about by the dog's defence system. The damage is not caused directly by the tick. The necrosis can be virtually eliminated by the prior destruction of polymorphonuclear leucocytes. (Polymorphonuclear leucocytes or polymorphs are blood cells which have a phagocytic role in the defence system.) Some allergic reactions to seemingly harmless agents result in tissue damage which is out of all proportion to the threat posed by the allergen. Hayfever can be very incapacitating and is the consequence of a reaction by our defence system to harmless, airborne pollen.

Clearly not all inflammatory reactions are useful. There is, for example, no obvious reason why the inflammatory reactions which occur in diseases such as rheumatic fever or rheumatoid arthritis benefit individuals. What is abundantly clear is that the combined effect of the components of the body's defensive mechanism may often be excessive. A study of inflammation tends to leave one with the distinct impression that the body generally overreacts to stimuli. If this is the case then we may be drawn to the view that inhibiting inflammatory reactions may in some circumstances be beneficial. Could it be that suppressing the inflammatory reactions associated with traumatic sports injuries falls into such a category?

Whilst there are many and varied kinds of inflammation, it is possible to consider that the basic components of the inflammatory reaction result from the combined effects of: changes in the microcirculation, alteration of permeability of the blood vessel walls to protein, and immigration of leucocytes and leucocyte-derived cells which exhibit activities such as phagocytosis.

## CHANGES IN THE MICROCIRCULATION DURING THE INFLAMMATORY RESPONSE

The immediate reaction of skin to a burn or irritant is to become reddened. This reddening will persist for a variable time depending on the severity of the stimulus. The redness is due to an increased volume of blood flowing through the inflamed area. Consequently the temperature of the inflamed skin rises and approaches that of the deep body temperature. This effect on the microcirculation is seen clearly if a firm line is drawn with a blunt point over a surface of the forearm. As Lewis demonstrated in 1927 a red line appears in the exact location of the stimulus. This dull red area is then surrounded by a bright red halo and a weal begins to form, first at the red line and then spreading outwards. Lewis confirmed earlier suggestions that many different types of injury could induce inflammation, including heat, cold, electric shock, radiation and chemical irritants, besides mechanical injury.

Detailed studies of vascular changes occurring during inflammation have been made by many physiologists who have observed vascular changes in sheets of living connective tissue arranged on microscope stages. Using this technique it is possible to observe mild inflammatory reactions over long periods of time. In this way it has been demonstrated that the whole capillary bed at the damaged site becomes suffused with blood at an increased pressure.

Capillaries dilate and many closed ones open up. The venules dilate and there is an increased flow of blood in the draining veins. This rapid flow gradually slows in the central capillaries and venules even though the vessels are still dilated. This slowing may gradually spread to the peripheral areas of the lesion and the flow may even stop completely. Despite this stasis the capillary pressure remains high, probably due to a resistance to outflow. Two of the cardinal signs of inflammation (heat and redness) are caused by this increase in blood flow to the affected area.

Another of the cardinal signs, swelling, is also the consequence of a change in the vascular system. In this case it is a change in the permeability of the blood vessel wall to protein. Normally the fluid found outside the blood system, in the tissues, is composed of water with some low-molecular-weight solutes such as sodium chloride. The protein content of this fluid is very low whilst the protein content of blood is relatively high. This state of affairs is maintained by virtue of the fact that the blood vessel wall is permeable only to water and salts. Proteins can not normally move from the blood vessel through the vessel wall into the surrounding tissues.

Water is forced out of small blood vessels at the arteriolar end of capillary beds due to the internal pressure that is generated by the pumping action of the heart on the blood, which is enclosed in the vascular system. The colloid osmotic pressure exerted by the protein present in the blood counterbalances this force causing water to be drawn back into the blood system. Without the presence of the plasma protein, blood volume would very rapidly diminish due to the net movement of water from the blood to the tissues.

During an inflammatory reaction the fluid equilibrium is altered. The permeability of small blood vessels changes to allow plasma protein to leak out of the vessel into the surrounding tissue. This change in distribution of protein is followed by a net passage of water from the blood into the tissues giving rise to the oedema, which may ultimately be seen as a swelling. Electron microscopic examination of blood vessels to which vasoactive substances were applied revealed the production of gaps 0.1-0.4 μm in diameter between adjacent endothelial cells. These gaps are temporary and there is no apparent damage caused to the endothelium of the leaking vessel.

Another consequence of oedema formation is the development of pain. Pain is, at least in part, due to the increased pressure on sensory nerves caused by the accumulation of the oedematous fluid. The common experience of relief that occurs instantly following the rupture of a painful boil lends itself to support this idea; there is, however, some evidence to support the idea that pain may also be due to the release of pain-inducing chemicals at the site of the reaction.

The cardinal signs of inflammation can thus be accounted for by the various changes that occur to the vasculature of the affected area. Vasodilatation results in the increased redness and temperature of the affected area whilst the change to the protein permeability of blood vessels results in the development of swelling and pain.

Even though each inflammatory reaction is unique, very similar reactions can be induced by widely differing stimuli. This has led to the idea that some intermediary control system exists to link the stimulus and the effect. The most popular idea is that the inflammatory insult activates or releases chemicals within the body, which then trigger the inflammatory reactions. This mediator concept was exemplified by Lewis, who proposed that the local vasodilatation and increased vascular permeability observed in the triple response could be mediated by a substance, liberated by the tissue, which he termed H-substance. The search for chemical mediators of inflammation has been particularly directed towards finding substances capable of increasing vascular permeability, largely because this parameter may be quantified quite easily.

It should be remembered, however, that mediators of increased vascular permeability might not necessarily be responsible for mediation of other aspects of the inflammatory reaction. The time course of vasodilatation and increased vascular permeability differ from each other markedly in many types of inflammatory reactions induced by chemical irritants. In general, investigations of permeability change mediation centre on endogenous substances which exhibit high permeability increasing potency and can be demonstrated in normal or inflamed tissues. Many such substances, including histamine and various metabolites of arachidonic acid, have been investigated to determine their possible role in the inflammatory responses.

## HISTAMINE

One of the first substances to be examined as a potential mediator of inflammation was histamine. Histamine is formed by the decarboxylation of the amino acid histidine and is a normal constituent of most tissues. The most abundant source of histamine in the body is to be found in the mast cells where it is stored in granules in association with the anti-coagulant substance heparin. Mast cells are found in high levels in the lungs, gastrointestinal system and skin. When released from the mast cell, or when injected, histamine produces vasodilatation and an increase in blood vessel permeability to protein. At high concentration histamine can also induce pain and so this particular locally acting hormone has the properties that could contribute to all four cardinal signs of inflammation.

Histamine has been found to be released following chemical, thermal, ionizing irradiation and immunological challenge. The contribution of histamine to most inflammatory reactions is limited, however, to the very early phase and in most cases, after the first few hours, anti-histamine drugs have no anti-inflammatory activity. The most notable exception is in the case of immunological reactions where histamine activity may persist throughout the reaction. In type I hypersensitivity reactions such as hayfever or urticaria, anti-histamine drugs represent an effective therapeutic approach throughout their duration.

## Arachidonic Acid Metabolites

Perhaps the most studied potential chemical mediators of inflammatory reactions are the various products of arachidonic acid metabolism. Every cell in the body has the capacity to generate some products from arachidonic acid, which is a 20-carbon, straight-chain, polyunsaturated fatty acid. This substance is usually found only at very low levels in the free form, but an abundant supply is normally available in a bound form, principally as cell membrane phospholipid. Following hormone activity or perturbation of the cell, the phospholipids are split by the action of enzymes such as phospholipase A2 causing the release of arachidonic acid and other, similar substrates. Once made available, arachidonic acid is metabolized in a way that is characteristic for the particular cell. This metabolism is generally rapid since it is the availability of arachidonic acid that is the rate-limiting factor. Two enzyme systems are available for this metabolism, a cyclooxygenase and a lipoxygenase. None of the biologically active products of these enzymes has a long half-life in the body and the products are not generally stored. They tend to exert their activities locally and it has become apparent that many of them exhibit opposing properties giving rise to the idea that they are involved in the local modulation of physiological processes.

The first class of these products to be discovered was the prostaglandins, so named because it was thought that they were secreted by the prostate gland, although it was subsequently found that the principal source of these substances (which are found in seminal fluid) was the seminal vesicles. Prostaglandins (PG) are formed by the action of the cyclo-oxygenase on arachidonic acid. This enzyme causes the oxygenation and internal cyclization of the fatty acid to give an unstable cyclic endoperoxide PGG2.

This unstable 15-hydroperoxy compound rapidly reduces to the 15-hydroxy derivative PGH2, this change being accompanied by the release of a free radical. It is worthy of mention here that free radicals are extremely damaging to biological tissues and may be responsible for some of the tissue destruction that occurs in the course of inflammatory reactions (free radicals are also generated by cells during phagocytosis). The second stage of synthesis involves another enzyme, which is tissue specific and results in the conversion of the cyclic endoperoxide to either PGE2, PGF2a, PGI or to a thromboxane depending on the tissue.

There appear to be two distinct cyclo-oxygenase enzymes, cyclo-oxygenase 1 and cyclo-oxygenase 2. The cyclo-oxygenase 1 is normally present in cells whilst the cyclo-oxygenase 2 appears to be an inducible enzyme which may have a very distinct role in the course of an inflammatory reaction.

Tremendous interest has been shown in these highly biologically active substances since the discovery of their presence in inflammatory exudates. Several properties exhibited by prostaglandins are compatible with the idea that these locally acting hormones are mediators of the inflammatory response. First, they can cause profound vasodilatation at very low concentrations and the erythema that they induce is very long lasting, persisting even after the prostaglandins have been broken down. Prostaglandins by themselves do not greatly affect vascular permeability nor do they evoke a pain response at physiological concentrations.

Prostaglandins do, however, radically enhance the vascular permeability increasing and pain-provoking activity of other substances such as histamine and bradykinin. These properties, coupled with the fact that raised prostaglandin levels are readily detectable in a number of inflammatory conditions, make them ideal candidates for the role of mediators of inflammation.

## LEUCOCYTES IN INFLAMMATION

Some types of inflammatory reaction such as acute allergic responses are restricted to changes in the microcirculation alone. More persistent inflammatory reactions of the type common to sports injuries, however, involve another major physiological change, that is the influx of leucocytes. The most significant leucocyte in the normal reaction to traumatic injury is the polymorph. There are several different kinds of polymorphs but the most abundant can be identified in a blood smear by virtue of their affinity to take up a neutral pH stain. These cells are sometimes referred to as neutrophils.

Normal tissues contain few extravascular polymorphs, but in an inflammatory reaction these cells may pass from the microcirculation into the damaged tissue site. Following an injury, blood polymorphs stick momentarily to the endothelium; they roll along the inside surface of the vessel wall, adhering briefly until they re-enter the circulation. After a few minutes, more and more cells adhere, and eventually these are not dislodged by the blood flow. In this way the endothelium comes to be lined with leucocytes, a process known as margination. Other leucocytes, platelets and red cells may also stick. Margination is promoted by the rapid deployment of selectins on the surface of the endothelial cells. Polymorphs have attachment sites on their cell surfaces for these selectins.

The marginated polymorphs leave the intravascular site by a process, which starts with a pseudopodium insinuating itself between two adjacent endothelial cells that form the blood vessel wall. The bulk of the polymorph, including the nucleus, then passes between the endothelial cells and comes to lie outside the endothelial cell but within the basement membrane. The cell then passes through the basement membrane.

These cells make an important contribution to the inflammatory process. The inflammatory response that occurs in experimental animals when their polymorphonuclear leucocytes have been depleted can be significantly reduced. To achieve this reduction the number of both circulating polymorphs and polymorphs that enter the circulation (presumably from the bone marrow) following an inflammatory stimulus must be reduced to very low levels. Polymorphonuclear leucocytes are the first inflammatory cells to accumulate in large numbers in an injured area.

These cells are phagocytic and play a protective role by ingesting and subsequently digesting invading micro-organisms or tissue debris in the affected area. Polymorphs do not survive for more than a few hours outside blood vessels and when they die they release their contents, which include lysosomal granules that contain a wide range of catabolic enzymes, into the surrounding area. These highly destructive enzymes may be responsible for additional damage occurring to the tissues.

As well as the influx of polymorphonuclear cells from the blood there is also a movement of mononuclear cells. Monocytes begin to move into the affected site at the same time as the polymorphs but they are slower and are therefore generally outnumbered by polymorphonuclear cells at the start of a reaction. Mononuclear cells are, however, much more enduring than the polymorphs and in many reactions begin to predominate after a day or so.

Outside of the circulation monocytes go through a maturation phase becoming macrophages which, as the name implies, are large phagocytic cells. These cells can undergo cell division, which also contributes to the large numbers of mononuclear cells that accumulate at the inflamed site.

Mononuclear cells such as macrophages do have a number of other, significant roles. They are capable of secreting many different chemicals that affect defensive activities and they have a key role in determining whether the body mounts an antibody-generating response to a challenge.

In the same way that changes in the microcirculation are brought about by chemical mediation the influx of leucocytes is also subject to chemical control. The simplest explanation of the phenomena of cell migration is that a chemical stimulus originating from the damaged site is recognized by leucocytes that respond by moving along a concentration gradient of the chemical towards the highest concentration. This process is called chemotaxis. There are a number of chemotactic substances known to be released from inflammatory sites and whilst cells may respond in a minor way to the mediators which affect changes in the vasculature the most potent agents have little effect on the microcirculation.

Arachidonic acid can be metabolized by a lipoxygenase enzyme system to generate a range of hydroxyeicosatetraenoic acids, one of which is 5,12-dihydroxyeicosatetraenoic acid or leukotriene B4 (LTB4). LTB4 is a potent chemotactic agent for polymorphonuclear leucocytes and mononuclear cells. LTB4 also stimulates the general activity of leucocytes as well as inducing more rapid movement and the release of destructive enzymes into the area. Thus when arachidonic acid is released from cell membranes the resultant prostaglandins and leukotrienes produced may, between them, mediate the development of all the major processes involved in an inflammatory response.

Another important source of chemotactic agents is the complement system. This is a complex system of plasma proteins that can be activated by a variety of stimuli including antigen-antibody interaction and endotoxin release to produce a powerful cytolytic, membrane-attack unit. Complement activation is an example of a biological cascade in which a small stimulus results in a large response. (The complement system has much in common with the blood-clotting cascade.) In the course of activation a number of small fragments, split off from complement components, are released into the area and some of these are powerfully chemotactic. Examples include components C3a and C5a, which are also potent histamine releasers and the aggregate C567 fraction. The complement system represents about 10 per cent of plasma protein and has been implicated in a variety of inflammatory reactions. Other chemotactic material can be released from the breakdown of the structural protein collagen and from the breakdown of the blood-clotting protein fibrin.

The contributions of the leucocytes to the inflammatory reactions are various. The presence of cells capable of phagocytosis at an injured site is an advantage. The removal of damaged tissues and any foreign material such as micro-organisms is of obvious importance. The local increase in leucocyte numbers at the site of inflammation results in a general increase in the concentration of proteolytic enzymes, because the lysosomes of the leucocytes contain cathepsins, hydrolases and other catabolic enzymes.

Release of these enzymes may be an important factor in the maintenance of inflammation by the production of altered tissue proteins and by the non-specific activation of thrombin, kinin and plasmin systems. Polymorphs also provide a source of enzymes with more specific activities for maintaining the inflammatory reaction. The release of kininogenases from polymorphs has been reported, and the presence of a specific collagenase in human polymorphs has been noted. Polymorphs may also contribute to the generation of prostaglandins in the inflammatory site.

## ACUTE AND CHRONIC INFLAMMATION

The initial reaction to most types of injury is an acute inflammatory response exhibiting the prominent feature of increased vascular permeability. This reaction will normally resolve in time and, if actual tissue necrosis is slight, no identifiable trace of the reaction will be left. In a more severe situation repair is effected by the synthesis of connective tissue to form a scar.

In some circumstances, however, inflammation may

persist. This chronic reaction may be caused by the presence of some foreign material that is not easily removed from the inflammatory site. It has been found that the resolution of an inflammatory lesion is invariably associated with the disappearance of the inflammatory-inducing irritant, but persistent inflammation may not necessarily be caused by any detectable irritant.

The aetiology of rheumatoid arthritis, for example, is uncertain. The characteristic feature of chronic inflammation is the presence of leucocytes at the site of reaction. Some acute inflammatory reactions may proceed without migration of phagocytic cells into the tissues, but chronic inflammation is invariably associated with large numbers of extravascular white cells. Chronic inflammation is also characterized by concurrent tissue destruction and resultant inflammation. The death of invading polymorphs at an inflamed site with the resultant release of all the cellular enzymes can give rise to a suppurative lesion. A suppurative lesion may continue at the site of some foreign material, but the necrotic area may become surrounded by a deposition of fibrous material and white cells to give rise to an abscess. A separation of degenerative and synthetic processes as in the case of an abscess is not always seen, the two processes often occurring simultaneously at the same site. Such a chronic inflammatory mass is called a granuloma.

Chronic inflammation can occur, however, without passing through an acute or suppurative phase by the gradual development of the chronic state. Histological examination of chronic inflammatory lesions reveals the presence of a variety of different types of white cell. In rheumatoid synovial fluids large numbers of white cells, principally polymorphs, can be found. These have extremely short half-lives of the order of only 3-4 hours and the variety of damaging agents which can be released from these cells has already been outlined. Polymorphs are also actively phagocytic, but this function may not be important in chronic inflammatory situations since their short life-span will frequently result in the release of any ingested material on the death of the cell. The predominant variety of polymorph is the neutrophil, but eosinophilic polymorphs, which share many of the properties of the neutrophil, also occur in inflammatory foci, possibly as a marker of general polymorph involvement, and in certain reactions the eosinophilic polymorph may predominate. Most chronic inflammatory reactions are characterized by the presence of large numbers of mononuclear cells.

Those mononuclear cells in a chronic inflammatory state may be derived either by emigration or division and the persistence of these cells may be due to their great longevity. Macrophages, like polymorphs, are phagocytic and this would seem to be an important function, the removal of foreign material and tissue debris being a prerequisite for the resolution of a reaction.

Within an area of chronic inflammation macrophages may be transformed into two other cell types: epithelioid cells and foreign body giant cells. Epithelioid cells are a common feature of granulomatous inflammation and can be transformed into epithelial cells by natural maturation if they live long enough, and do not have undigested phagocytosed material within the cell. Giant cells are multinucleate and have been shown to be produced by cell fusion, although this fusion may be followed by nuclear division without cytoplasmic fission.

These cells are found in large numbers around foreign bodies that are too large for macrophages to engulf. Other cells present in chronic inflammatory reactions are fibroblasts, which are probably derived from local connective tissue fibroblasts and are responsible for collagen deposition, and lymphocytes and plasma cells, which are responsible for the production of antibodies that facilitate the elimination of micro-organisms.

Our knowledge of inflammatory processes has largely been derived from observations made in humans with chronic inflammatory disease and in laboratory experiments in animals. The contribution that any of the factors described above may make in the inflammatory sequel to a sporting injury cannot be specified but undoubtedly there will be several predictable phenomena.

- An influx of blood giving rise to the characteristic heat and redness.
- A movement of plasma protein and associated water into the tissue, causing swelling.
- An influx of phagocytic cells that have the potential to cause tissue destruction.
- Pain, due perhaps to pressure on the nerve endings caused by the swelling or to the effect of chemical mediators of pain being released.

5. Finally, and perhaps most importantly to the sportsman, there will be a loss of function-Virchow's fifth cardinal sign.

The persistence of the problem depends on many factors, but certainly the influx of leucocytes and the release of their enzyme-rich content may compound the damage already caused and tend to prolong the duration of the reaction. Given that no further aggravation occurs and that there are no complications, resolution should occur within days or weeks and at worst months.

A pertinent question to ask at this point is whether the inflammation that follows a traumatic injury is necessary. Clearly the body automatically takes what it deems to be the safest course of action when injured. It directs its defensive systems to the area to make sure that no microbial invasion occurs and that all the necessary resources are made available to repair the damage. It is evident, however, that the body has a tendency to overreact. The response in many cases may be more serious than the stimulus.

## THE TREATMENT OF SPORTING INJURIES

The acronym 'RICE' will be familiar to those with experience of treating sports injuries. Rest, ice, compression and elevation are all of value. Rest enables healing and limits adding to the damage already sustained. Applying pressure to an affected area and the elevation of a limb above the level of the heart can influence the intravascular-extravascular fluid balance equilibrium with a resultant inhibition of oedema development.

Cooling a traumatized part of the body is also effective.

A common sight these days is the arrival on the field of play of the trainer who reaches into his bag for the aerosol can with which he sprays some area of the prostrated participant being attended. The injured player stands gingerly and then cautiously runs on. The trainer collects up the bag with its 'magic' spray and walks off. These aerosol sprays contain volatile compounds that evaporate on the skin surface causing rapid chilling of the area.

The practice of cooling an injured area whether by volatile spray, cold compress or ice-packs, if applied rapidly, may well reduce the immediate response to minor trauma by inhibiting the active processes which are involved in the initiation of an inflammatory reaction. Problems have arisen because of the abuse of these solvent-based products for 'sniffing'. Nevertheless cooling will undoubtedly reduce the immediate reaction to a traumatic stimulus. Given that the body does seem to have a natural inclination to overreact, inducing a delay in the response produced by cooling may well prevent, or at least limit, any subsequent inflammation.

Other non-specific topical applications that can be used successfully for the treatment of injured tissues include liniments. These preparations are rubefacients and are thought to act by counter-irritation. This is a phenomenon where mild or moderate pain can be relieved by irritating the skin. Counter-irritation is effective in providing relief from painful lesions of muscles, tendons and joints. There is, however, little evidence that the topical application of preparations containing adrenaline or aspirin is of value in the relief of pain.

A number of more specific, anti-inflammatory treatments are available to deal with sporting injuries. The reduction of pain and inflammation represents an obvious therapeutic target. It is clear, however, that great care must be taken in judging the severity of an injury. Pain is the cue that intimates the severity of a problem. There are many drugs which can reduce our appreciation of pain, but a reduction of pain sensation may lead to the induction of further damage to an injury by the failure to respond to the natural inclination to rest. Clear evidence of the dangers of masking pain sensation can be seen amongst those who suffer the peripheral mutilation common amongst people with impaired sensory nerve activity such as that which occurs in untreated leprosy victims. Anti-inflammatory drugs may nevertheless be of value.

## THE USE OF ANTI-INFLAMMATORY DRUGS TO TREAT INFLAMMATORY CONDITIONS

Although the treatment of inflammation with anti-inflammatory agents was practised by Hippocrates, who recommended the chewing of willow bark for a variety of ailments, such sensible practices were largely forgotten during subsequent centuries. It was not until 1876 that a physician named MacLagan revolutionized the treatment of rheumatic fever (and, indeed, other inflammatory conditions) by the reintroduction of an extract of willow bark called salicin. MacLagan had been unimpressed with the treatments that were routinely used to treat rheumatic fever (a condition characterized by extensive inflammatory lesions) which even included such measures as blood letting.

A synthetic analogue of this glycoside was soon produced and in 1899 a German pharmaceutical company, Bayer, introduced a more palatable derivative, acetylsalicylic acid under the trade name Aspirine. Over 100 years later we still have aspirin readily available as a simple, cheap and effective remedy for a wide variety of ailments. It has been the subject of innumerable clinical trials in many diverse areas of medicine ranging from the treatment of food intolerance to the prevention of heart attacks. Without doubt though, the bulk of the tens of thousands of tons of aspirin consumed each year is taken for the alleviation of pain, inflammation and fever.

Since the introduction of aspirin many other drugs with similar therapeutic profiles have been developed and there are now about 20 aspirin-like drugs available for clinical use in the UK, although only aspirin and ibuprofen are available for general purchase. These aspirin-like drugs, generally referred to collectively as non-steroidal anti-inflammatory drugs or NSAIDs, all have proven anti-inflammatory activity in the treatment of chronic inflammatory conditions such as rheumatoid arthritis. Countless clinical trials have demonstrated the efficacy of these agents in alleviating both objective and subjective symptoms of inflammatory disease. Whilst some of these agents are more popular than others, there is no clear indication that any particular example is more effective than the others.

Indeed it is difficult to find convincing proof that any of the newer drugs in this class is more effective than aspirin. The assessment of activity of this type of drug is, however, fraught with difficulties. It is not easy to find large numbers of patients with similar disease states who are prepared to be subjected to the withdrawal of their effective therapy so that they may be used as controls in such trials. It is also very difficult to quantify a reduction in inflammation.

Given that these difficulties exist when testing drugs on common chronic conditions, it is not hard to appreciate that the difficulties involved in testing anti-inflammatory agents in acute sporting injuries, which may affect any part of the body, are considerably greater. Since a chronically inflamed joint in a patient with rheumatoid arthritis may remain in a similar condition for weeks on end, the effect of introduction and withdrawal of an effective anti-inflammatory agent on the level of inflammation of that joint should be seen fairly easily.

A traumatic sporting injury should progressively heal over a fairly limited period without intervention. How then can you measure the efficacy of an anti-inflammatory drug superimposed on a naturally regressing inflammatory condition? The simple answer is with great difficulty!

The majority of clinical trials published on the efficacy of aspirin-like drugs in sports injury are organized with two groups of injured subjects. One group is treated with one example of a NSAID whilst the other group is treated with a different NSAID. The usual result of these trials is that no significant difference is established between the two drugs under test. Clinical trials using this protocol are usually used to establish that a new NSAID is effective.

The trial protocol makes the assumption that the older, perhaps more established drug is, itself, effective. This assumption may not be valid and, if it is not, then the trial does not produce reliable results.

Whilst NSAIDs are clearly effective in the treatment of chronic disease, evidence that they do have a role to play in acute traumatic injury treatment is much more limited. To establish definitively that drugs can treat a sports injury effectively a number of criteria have to be met. First, suitable injuries, preferably all of a certain type, would be needed in reasonable numbers. Second, some measure of effectiveness would be required which is meaningful.

Third, a comparison would have to be made with a group of similar patients receiving no active treatment, that is, a control group. Because many individuals are responsive to suggestion, subjects in the control group would have to receive what appears to be the same treatment as the test group but, of course, without the active drug. In other words one group would be given tablets containing the drug whilst the other group would be given identical-looking tablets but with no drug in them, so-called placebos.

Now with regard to the first two criteria, perhaps a good place to look for a plentiful supply of similar sports injuries would be in a club where members are involved in the same sport with, therefore, the same injury tendencies. A measurement of the period of time following injury until the injured person is fit for competition or full training again could serve as the key to assess effectiveness. If this time is reduced in the drug-treated group then it could be concluded that the drug is a successful therapy. With regard to the third criterion, however, there is a substantial ethical and moral problem. If the drug works or even if it is thought to work, it is difficult to justify the withholding of that treatment for the purpose of a trial since this action might unnecessarily prolong the period of absence from the sport. In many professional clubs such an action would be unacceptable.

## THE MECHANISM OF ACTION OF ANTI-INFLAMMATORY DRUGS

Despite the relative paucity of convincing trials that

demonstrate the effectiveness of these anti-inflammatory drugs, their use in the treatment of sports injuries is very widespread. The commencement of a course of NSAIDs immediately after the injury occurs appears to be an effective way to reduce the recovery time. The most commonly used drugs in this class are aspirin, diclofenac, ibuprofen, indomethacin, naproxen and piroxicam.

The use of these drugs, though widespread, remains largely empirical, as there is no universally accepted explanation of how they reduce inflammation. Indeed our understanding of the processes involved in soft tissue injury is far from complete. Several suggestions have been made, however, to explain the antiinflammatory activity of the aspirin-like drugs. Considerable attention has been focused on the possible interaction of these drugs with various factors involved in this inflammatory process.

For example, many early attempts to explain the anti-inflammatory activity of these drugs considered their ability to interfere with proteolytic enzymes. These enzymes are involved both in the early stages of inflammation and in the later stages when the process is well established. An inhibition of proteolytic enzyme activity either at the start of the reaction, preventing the activation of the complement, kinin, fibrin or plasmin systems, or during the later, autocatabolic stage of inflammation could be the mechanism of action. Certainly many antiinflammatory drugs have been shown to have some measure of anti-protease activity, but the general correlation between enzyme inhibition and antiinflammatory activity is not impressive.

Aspirin derivatives are known to inhibit a large number of enzyme systems, but inhibition is generally seen only at drug concentrations that exceed the normal therapeutic level. Another explanation that has been proposed which is closely related to this idea is that the anti-inflammatory drugs reduce inflammation by preventing the release of enzymes from lysosomes during the more established phase of the reaction. Again, whilst there is some experimental evidence available to support this idea, overall, it is not a convincing explanation.

With an improved understanding of the mediation of inflammation came the idea that the action of anti-inflammatory drugs might be due to an interference with the activities of one or more of the proposed chemical mediators of inflammation. It was not, however, until 1971 that any major headway was made in this area of our understanding. In a series of three papers published in Nature.

John Vane and his colleagues outlined the hypothesis that the action of the aspirin-like drugs could be attributed to their ability to suppress the synthesis of prostaglandins. Virtually all NSAIDs have been shown to inhibit the synthesis of prostaglandins and they generally exhibit this property at concentrations that are low enough to be achieved with normal therapeutic doses of the drugs.

The predictable consequences of the inhibition of prostaglandin synthesis on an inflammatory process (based on the known pro-inflammatory activities of the prostaglandins) easily lead us to the conclusion that this property of NSAIDs provides an explanation for their mechanisms of action.

A reduction in the level of prostaglandins at an inflammatory site should result in a reduction in the symptoms of heat and redness since prostaglandins would normally promote an increased blood flow to the area by virtue of their ability to cause profound erythema. A reduction in the pain associated with the reaction could also be anticipated, since, in the absence of prostaglandins, there would be no state of hyperalgesia. In other words the tissue would not exhibit a greater sensitivity to painful stimuli than normal. Oedema would also be reduced in severity as the permeability-increasing effect of chemical agents on blood vessel walls would not be subject to the normal exaggerating action of the prostaglandins.

Thus we can see that the reduction in synthesis of the prostaglandins that can be demonstrated when using NSAIDs could account for the reduction of all the cardinal signs of inflammation. As additional support for this idea of a single, common mechanism of action for NSAIDs, other properties exhibited by this group of drugs can also be explained by an inhibition of prostaglandin synthesis. For example, as well as being analgesic, antiinflammatory drugs, these compounds are invariably anti-pyretic agents as well, that is they have the ability to reduce elevated body temperature.

During fever prostaglandins are detectable in increased quantities in the cerebrospinal fluid which fills the cavities of the brain, and it has been shown in animals that the injection of prostaglandins into the anterior hypothalamus evokes a pyrexic response. The inhibition of prostaglandin synthesis, therefore, offers an explanation for this property of these drugs, in addition to their anti-inflammatory action.

Another property, which is common to most of these agents, is that they inhibit platelet aggregation. To repair damaged blood vessels, platelets come together to form a plug to fill the gap and prevent bleeding. This activity is in part mediated via the synthesis of thromboxanes by the platelets. Drugs such as aspirin, which inhibits the cyclo-oxygenase enzyme, will prevent the synthesis, not only of prostaglandins but of thromboxanes as well, preventing normal platelet function. In some circumstances, notably when there is already some impairment to normal platelet function, this activity of these drugs may represent a hazard. There is, however, much interest in the use of this anti-platelet activity to prevent the development of thrombosis. Small blood clot fragments may lodge in the vascular beds of the brain or heart and a very small regular dose of aspirin may protect a subject from a stroke or a heart attack.

Another common feature of NSAIDs is their tendency to cause gastric irritation and this, too, can be explained by a mechanism of prostaglandin synthesis inhibition. Prostaglandins normally limit the amount of hydrochloric acid secreted by the parietal cells in the main gastric glands, probably by an action on the enzyme adenylate cyclase. In addition, prostaglandins may promote the functional vasodilatation necessary for the parietal cells in their secretory mode. If the levels of prostaglandins in the stomach are reduced then a greater amount of acid will be secreted and this acid will be produced by cells that have been forced into this synthetic activity without the usual increased provision of oxygen. This situation may thus result in a gastritis in which some mucosal tissue may be damaged by the ischaemia that can result from the increased metabolic activity occurring without increased blood flow.

We do, therefore, have a proposed mechanism of action for NSAIDs that can be invoked to explain not only their anti-inflammatory activity, but also their anti-pyretic and anti-platelet activities. The proposition even serves to explain their most common side-effect. This brief account of mechanism would be less than complete, however, if it did not at least indicate one or two of the many observations that have been reported which do not easily fit within this explanation.

First, sodium salicylate is some 100 times less effective than acetylsalicylate (aspirin) as an inhibitor of prostaglandin synthesis whereas they are of similar anti-inflammatory activity. Secondly, in experiments in which inflammation has been induced in essential fatty acid-deficient animals (i.e. animals rendered incapable of generating prostaglandins) aspirin has been shown to be as effective at reducing inflammation as it is in normal animals. As a final example of the type of observation that is not compatible with this theory it has been shown that even small sub-anti-inflammatory doses of aspirin render the inflamed synovial tissue of arthritic joints incapable of producing prostaglandins for several days. Clearly, however compelling the idea that inhibition of prostaglandin synthesis is the explanation for the mechanism of action of aspirin, an explanation is required as to why regular high doses of the drug are needed to achieve an anti-inflammatory action when two or three tablets, two or three times a week would seem to be all that is necessary to induce effective inhibition of prostaglandin synthesis.

The relationship between prostaglandin synthesis and the NSAIDs is, thus, confused. On the one hand we have a convincing and attractive hypothesis which explains the many and varied activities and even side-effects of this group of drugs by one, simple and elegant mechanism. On the other hand we have evidence that not all anti-inflammatory drugs are good inhibitors of prostaglandin synthesis, that aspirin can exert an anti-inflammatory effect in the absence of any prostaglandin synthesis and that it is too good at inhibiting prostaglandin synthesis in rheumatic patients to explain why such large amounts of the drug are needed in clinical practice.

## NSAIDS IN SPORTS INJURY

Whatever the mechanism by which these drugs exert their effect, their use in the treatment of chronic inflammatory disease is well established and their efficacy beyond question. Similarly in the treatment of acute traumatic injury their use has become commonplace and although far too many clinical trails have failed to furnish proof of their efficacy, clear evidence that these drugs are of benefit in sports injury has been produced. These drugs represent a simple and relatively safe means of reducing the inflammatory response to an injury. They may also help to return an injured sports participant to competitive fitness more rapidly. Many clinical trials compare the use of two different anti-inflammatory drugs but the most common finding is that there is no significant difference between the two. Where differences are reported they are not consistent. It would therefore be difficult to indicate a rank order of efficacy for these drugs.

Sprains strains (partial tearing of muscles) and bruises are all painful examples of sports injuries. Commonly they may warrant the use of painkilling (analgesic) drugs such as paracetamol or even in severe cases a narcotic analgesic compound such as dihydrocodeine. Since, however, these conditions are generally associated with an inflammatory component the use of an analgesic drug with antiinflammatory activity would seem to be a more logical choice. About twenty different NSAIDs are available which could be used to treat sports injuries and some details are given here of a small selection of them.

### Aspirin

Aspirin is a very effective analgesic drug at a dose of 2-3

g per day. At higher doses, that is in excess of 4 g per day, aspirin will reduce the swelling of an inflamed joint, a property not shown at the lower, analgesic level. Whilst anti-inflammatory activity is seen only at higher doses it is inadvisable to exceed the normal recommended doses without qualified medical supervision.

Despite the antiquity of this preparation, unequivocal evidence that any of the newer challengers offers an all-round superior performance is lacking. The general availability, and low cost of aspirin make it an ideal candidate for self-treatment following sports injury. Aspirin use is, however, not devoid of side-effects, although the risks involved with the use of the drug are probably generally overstated. Given that the injured athlete is an otherwise normal, healthy adult, the major problem liable to be encountered following the use of aspirin (or indeed, for that matter, any of the NSAIDs) is gastric irritation which may be experienced as a form of dyspepsia.

Attempts to reduce this problem by modifying the tablets in a variety of ways have not been particularly successful. It is now generally recognized that the effect of these drugs on the stomach is due not so much to the unabsorbed drug in contact with the gastric mucosa as to the effect of the drug after its absorption. The most effective way to minimize this problem is to avoid the use of these drugs when the stomach is empty. If the drugs are taken following a meal then any increased acid production that ensues can be utilized in the digestive process rather than being free to attack the lining of the stomach itself.

In 1984 Anderson and Gotzsche compared the use of aspirin and another NSAID, naproxen, in patients with sports injuries. Perhaps not surprisingly, they found no significant differences between the two drugs. Whilst this type of trial is common and the finding typical, the authors did highlight a phenomenon very relevant to the treatment of this type of traumatic injury. They demonstrated that significantly better results were obtained when the interval between injury and the start of treatment was shorter. This effect is widely appreciated now and is exactly what would be predicted from experimental inflammation studies in animals. In laboratory tests of the type used to screen for anti-inflammatory activity of new drugs for the treatment of arthritis it can be shown clearly that NSAIDs are much more effective against developing inflammation than they are against established inflammation.

The implications of this are clear. If it is deemed necessary to use an antiinflammatory drug to treat a sports injury, it should be given as early as possible after the damage is sustained and certainly before the inflammation becomes established. The principal reason for this probably lies in the realm of the intravascular/extravascular fluid equilibrium. The role of permeability changes has already been highlighted. Protein moves through the blood vessel wall during the development of the inflammatory reaction and draws water with it resulting in the oedematous swelling. Once this oedema is formed, its resolution is dependent on the removal of the extravascular protein. NSAIDs do not appear to have any effect on the extravascular protein. It is an inevitable conclusion, therefore, that preventing oedema development is easier than resolving established oedema as there is no mechanism for the rapid removal of this protein for the resolution of an established reaction.

## Naproxen

Naproxen is one of the mainstays of treatment for chronic inflammatory conditions. Its efficacy and safety record are excellent and it is one of the most frequently prescribed drugs for the treatment of arthritis. Since its introduction in the early 1970s naproxen has been the subject of a large number of trials in the treatment of soft tissue injuries. Whilst many of these compare naproxen with another NSAID and find no difference in activity, several trials have shown naproxen to be better than the other drug in some respects and naproxen has been shown to be superior to placebo.

In view of the popularity of this drug and the generally good reports of its efficacy in the literature, naproxen must rank high amongst the most suitable drugs for the treatment of sporting injuries. The drug is given at a dose of 0.75-1.25 g per day in 3 or 4 divided doses. Initially a high loading dose of 500 mg may be given to aid the rapid attainment of suitable plasma levels of the drug (750 μg/ml). The drug may be taken at meal times to help combat any gastric discomfort felt, although in the presence of food the drug is absorbed more slowly. More rapid absorption occurs with the use of naproxen sodium. A 500 mg naproxen suppository preparation is available, principally for use at night.

## Ibuprofen

Ibuprofen is another NSAID with a similar structure to naproxen. It is the oldest propionic acid derivative anti-inflammatory agent in use and considerable experience has, therefore, been obtained with it. This drug is also one of the few drugs of this class available in the UK without prescription. It has a reputation for being well tolerated. In other words, it is widely felt that this particular anti-inflammatory agent does not induce the same degree of dyspepsia as many of its rivals. In the UK, the Committee on Safety of Medicines (CSM) advises that ibuprofen is associated with the lowest risk of serious upper gastrointestinal side-effects of seven oral NSAIDs reviewed. The other NSAIDs considered by the CSM were piroxicam, ketoprofen, indomethacin, naproxen and diclofenac which were considered to be associated with intermediate risk and azapropazone which was considered to be associated with the highest risk.

Ibuprofen has always been perceived to be a well-tolerated drug. It is possible, however, that much of its reputation is based on early experiences with the drug when it was used at relatively low dose levels. To improve the often disappointing activity of ibuprofen the doses used have been increased and whilst the drug is still generally well tolerated it is certainly not without gastric irritant activity at these higher levels. Trials using ibuprofen at doses as low as 1200 mg per day have been shown to reduce pain and recovery time of soft-tissue sports injuries. Trials have, however, tended to use higher doses than this. Hutson found no significant differences between the activity of ibuprofen given at doses of 1.8 or 2.4 g daily amongst 46 patients with sporting injuries to the knee. The normal recommended dose range for ibuprofen for musculoskeletal disorders is 1.2-1.8 g daily in 3 or 4 divided doses, preferably after food. This may be increased if necessary to the maximum recommended daily dose of 2.4 g.

## Indomethocin

Indomethacin has been used for treating inflammatory conditions since the mid-1960s and remains a very frequently prescribed drug. Whilst being an effective anti-inflammatory drug it does suffer, apart from the gastric irritant activity somewhat typical of this type of drug, from a number of central nervous system side-effects such as headaches, dizziness and light-headedness. Generally, indomethacin is found to be of similar efficacy to other NSAIDs, such as naproxen, in the treatment of soft-tissue sports injuries.

As might be expected, the drop-out rate due to side-effects of this drug is generally higher than for other members of this group of drugs with normal therapeutic doses of indomethacin (50-200 mg daily). The drug is normally initiated as 25 mg 2 or 3 times daily and gradually increased if necessary. Edwards et al. found it necessary to withdraw only one patient from a group of 53 who were receiving 75 mg of indomethacin daily for acute soft-tissue sports injuries. It is possible that at this low starting dose toxicity is less of a problem.

Indomethacin is also available in 100 mg suppositories for night-time use and these may be of benefit in some individuals. It should be remembered that the combined rectal and oral doses should not amount to more than 200 mg in a 24-hour period.

## Piroxicam

Piroxicam appears to be comparable with indomethacin or naproxen in treating acute musculoskeletal injuries and it is generally well tolerated. One particular advantage of piroxicam is that it has a long half-life, which permits its use as a single daily dose, usually of 20 mg. An initial, loading dose of 40 mg on each of the first 2 days of treatment, reducing to 20 mg for subsequent days may be used for acute musculoskeletal disorders.

In a large study of acute sports injuries in Norway the authors concluded that piroxicam at 40 mg daily for the first 2 days and 20 mg daily for a further 5 days resulted in significant improvements in mobility and reductions in pain when compared with placebo (Lereim and Gabor, 1988). This treatment gave a marginally superior response when compared with naproxen at 500 mg twice daily, and both drugs were well tolerated.

Piroxicam may also be given as a deep intramuscular injection for the initial dose. Effective concentrations of drugs are usually achieved earlier in this way than when they are administered orally.

### Diclofenac

Diclofenac is another useful drug of this class. Available in both 75 and 100 mg tablets, daily doses of 75-150 mg are recommended. In a trial involving subjects with severely sprained ankles, diclofenac at 150 mg daily was shown to be superior to both placebo and piroxicam at 20 mg daily. Both drugs were well tolerated. One possible advantage of this drug is that it is available in a slow-release form that is administered once daily, although this may be less of an advantage in the acute situation. In general, therapeutic levels are not achieved as rapidly with drugs that have a long half-life. Drugs with a short duration of action will normally give therapeutic levels in a very short period of time.

### Phenylbutazone

Phenylbutazone was introduced into clinical medicine in 1949 to take its place alongside the salicylates for the treatment of arthritic conditions. It is a powerful anti-inflammatory drug and is capable of treating acute exacerbations of rheumatoid arthritis and severe ankylosing spondylitis (an inflammatory condition of the spine). Compared with the many, newer antiinflammatory agents now available it is subject to a large number of toxic side-effects, some of which have led to fatal outcomes. Whilst many physicians believe this to be an extraordinarily useful anti-inflammatory agent, others have argued that it is too dangerous to use.

The most serious side-effects are undoubtedly the retention of fluid which in predisposed individuals may precipitate cardiac failure, and the interference with normal blood cell production, most commonly resulting in aplastic anaemia and agranulocytosis which can occur within the first few days of treatment. Its use, therefore, in self-limiting musculoskeletal disorders is difficult to justify. In the UK phenylbutazone is now only indicated for the treatment of ankylosing spondylitis in hospital situations. In the past it has been somewhat abused, particularly in the United States. A report by Marshall indicates that in the National Football League, for example, an average of 24-40 unit doses of phenylbutazone was used per player per season.

Whatever the role of phenylbutazone in injuries in sportsmen and women, there is no doubt that this drug has been used considerably in the field of equestrian sports. In show jumping the horses' feet are subjected to constant concussion. By the age of 10 many show-jumping horses will have suffered pathological changes in their feet but in many cases will be at their peak.

Similarly 3-day event horses are subject to considerable physical stress, with strain of a tendon or the suspensory ligament being common injuries. Even without jumping-related competition, the regular galloping activity, as in for example, flat racing or polo, may result in substantial changes in bones, joints and ligaments of a horse. When pushed too hard or for too long lameness may develop due to the pain and inflammation caused. The time-honoured remedy for reducing the pain and inflammation of these injuries in horses is to administer an anti-inflammatory drug, the most frequently used example being phenylbutazone.

Horses generally tolerate phenylbutazone very well and may be treated with the drug to improve their comfort. Whilst there are many indications for the use of phenylbutazone in horses, dilemmas do arise as to whether their use may mask an injury and lead to a complete breakdown of an affected limb. The governing bodies of equestrian sports generally recognize the usefulness of this drug but exclude the use of the drug on, or immediately before, competition days in order that no unfair advantage may be gained by improving performance and also to protect unfit horses from being used competitively.

### Rofecoxib and Celecoxib

These new NSAIDs are notable for their selective inhibition of the inducible cyclo-oxygenase 2. They are not currently licensed for the treatment of acute musculoskeletal disorders. If the ability to inhibit the cyclo-oxygenase enzyme selectively is advantageous for the treatment of acute inflammatory problems then these drugs may prove to be valuable in the future.

## DURATION OF NSAID TREATMENT

There are obvious advantages to the early treatment of inflammatory responses to injury. How long treatment should continue is less clear. Studies of NSAID treatment of soft tissue injuries in animals have generally demonstrated the advantage of treatment in the early, post-injury stage. The effectiveness of treatment over longer periods is less apparent. Some sports injuries studies have also reported no differences between treated and untreated groups at later stages of the inflammatory and healing processes.

In self-limiting injuries healing will generally occur without treatment. It is perhaps inevitable that differences between treated and non-treated groups will diminish with time. Whilst treatment may result in earlier return to normality, untreated subjects are likely to 'catch up'. There is, however, an alternative interpretation, which is that NSAIDs may actually slow down the healing process.

Inhibiting the influx of inflammatory cells, particularly polymorphonuclear leucocytes, may limit the amount of local tissue injury that occurs following trauma. It is possible that this may lead to the slower removal of damaged tissue and a consequent delay in the resolution of the injury. The production of scar tissue may be impaired if fibroblast activity is reduced and this could, indeed, reduce the speed at which fully functional tissues are reformed.

There is no consistent evidence that NSAIDs delay healing and, in consequence, explanations of possible mechanisms are largely speculative. Whilst sports injuries studies with NSAIDs do not universally demonstrate efficacy, the majority do. It would, therefore, seem to be a reasonable approach to treat acute traumatic sporting injuries immediately with NSAIDs but to discontinue treatment as soon as it is apparent that the acute inflammatory problem is resolving.

**Table.** Commonly Available Topical Preparations

| | |
|---|---|
| Piroxicam | Feldene |
| Ibuprofen | Fenbid Forte Gel, Ibugel, Ibumousse, Ibuspray, Proflex |
| Ketoprofen | Oruvail, Powegel |
| Felbinac | Traxam |
| Diclofenac | Voltarol |

## TOPICAL NSAIDS IN SPORTS INJURY

Several pharmaceutical companies produce topical preparations of NSAIDs for the relief of musculoskeletal pain. Topical preparations of salicylates, piroxicam, ibuprofen, ketoprofen, felbinac (the active metabolite of fenbufen) and diclofenac are currently available in the UK. The concept of applying a NSAID locally in an effort to maximize the level of the drug at the site of injury whilst minimizing the systemic level of the drug is an interesting one. In theory this technique may achieve a good therapeutic effect without the troublesome gastrointestinal side-effects sometimes encountered with systemic therapy.

There is good evidence that these preparations afford good penetration of the drug through the skin and that high levels of the active drug are achieved in the underlying tissues. Clinical trials with these preparations generally demonstrate that active drug formulations are more effective than placebo, but the differences are generally slight. In one celebrated double-blind study patients suffering bilateral inflammatory knee joint effusions were treated with diclofenac gel to one knee and a placebo gel to the other. It was found that there were small reductions in swelling in both knees and no significant difference between the drug-treated and placebo-treated knees could be detected. In other words it did not seem to matter which knee the NSAID was applied to!

It has been suggested that the massage of an affected area with a gel or cream may in itself be beneficial irrespective of the presence of a NSAID. A significant point which should be considered here is whether these compounds actually exert their anti-inflammatory action at the inflamed site or elsewhere. If, for example, the reality of the situation is that the drugs reduce inflammation by interacting in some way with components in the bloodstream, then the concept of local application would be flawed

## Proteolytic Enzymes as Anti-inflammatory Agents

Several reports have been published suggesting that proteolytic enzyme preparations are useful for the treatment of soft-tissue sports injuries. Hyaluronidase, which splits the glucosaminidic bonds of hyaluronic acid, reduces the viscosity of the cellular cement.

Local injections of this enzyme have been shown to reduce healing time of sprained ankles. Chymotrypsin preparations, which are available in tablet form, have also been found to be useful in sporting injuries. Whilst these enzymes are obviously vulnerable to gastrointestinal breakdown, there is evidence that some active enzyme is absorbed. A number of clinical trials have been conducted amongst professional soccer players and whilst not all have shown favourable results, some trials have found significant reductions in the recovery time to match fitness.

This is particularly the case when a haematoma or sprain is the major feature of the injury. In one notable trial an enzyme preparation was compared with placebo in injured footballers of a London club. The physicians monitoring the trial were so impressed by the apparent efficacy of the enzyme that the trial was abandoned since it was considered unjustifiable to withhold the enzyme from the placebo group. This was deemed especially so since the club was in the running for major honours in that season! Here though we have an enigma. On the one hand we have apparently convincing reports that proteolytic enzyme preparations aid recovery from sports injury. On the other hand we are faced with the fact that the bulk of these reports are over 30 years old.

If these preparations could significantly reduce recovery time and return players to match fitness in perhaps only 70 per cent of the normal time it should take, why are they not in use? Perhaps the optimistic initial findings have not been reproducible on subsequent occasions or perhaps toxicity has limited their use; it is true that occasionally serious hypersensitivity reactions do occur when administering high molecular weight substances such as enzymes. Whilst they are not used now for treating mechanically induced trauma, these preparations are regularly used in a variety of post-surgical situations to reduce oedema.

## Anti-inflammatory Steroids

Many of the body's natural hormones are based on the four-ring steroid structure. The precise activity of a steroid depends on which of a small number of substitutions are made to the structure. Some steroids (oestrogens, progesterones and testosterones) have powerful effects on sex-related attributes and activities. Others, such as the glucocorticoids or mineralocorticoids, influence the metabolic activities or fluid balance of the body.

The activities of steroids are seldom completely specific and often overlap each other. Of interest here are the most powerful anti-inflammatory agents known to humankind, the glucocorticoids. These are drugs that are based on the chemical structure of the steroids produced by the cortex of the adrenal gland and are generally referred to as corticosteroids. These corticosteroids were first used to treat inflammatory conditions in the late 1940s.

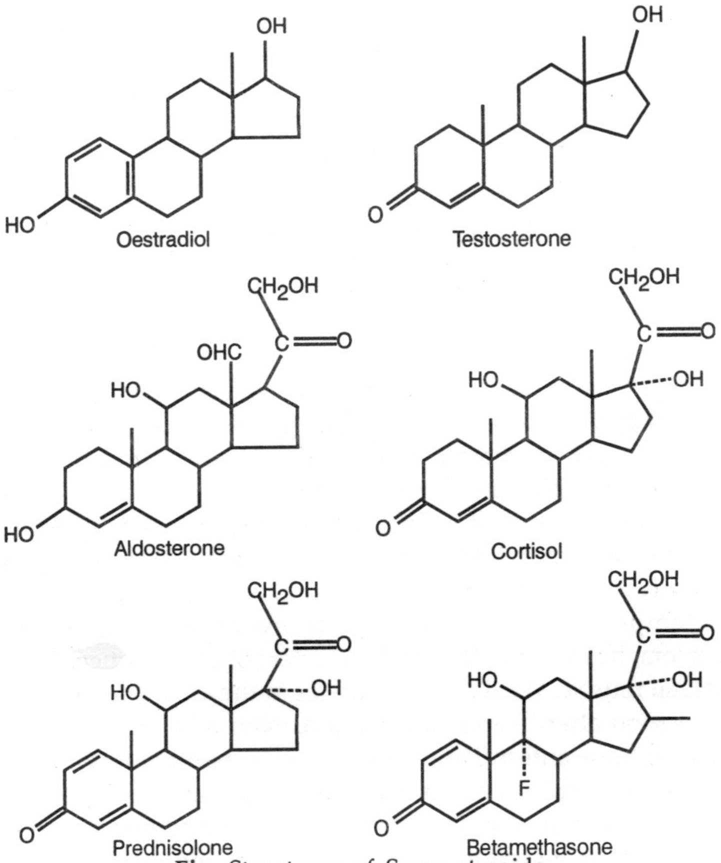


**Fig.** Structures of Some steroids.

They represented an exciting and, possibly, fundamental new approach to the treatment of inflammatory disease. Initial optimism waned rapidly, however, as it quickly became apparent that these substances were not curative and that they were subject to considerable numbers of side-effects. The anti-inflammatory activity of these steroid hormones appears to be secondary to their glucocorticoid function, as despite the severe metabolic derangement which accompanies adrenal gland insufficiency there is no general precipitation of inflammatory reactions. Many attempts have been made to increase the anti-inflammatory activity of these steroids. A large number of anti-inflammatory steroids are now available, many of which are an order of magnitude more potent than cortisol. All of these steroids have significant glucocorticoid activity.

Inevitably, long-term use of these drugs will affect the general metabolic activity of the body and is likely to provoke symptoms similar to those seen when the adrenal cortex is hyperactive (Cushing's syndrome). It is, therefore, important that a distinction is made between the long-term use of anti-inflammatory steroids and their use in acute situations. The long-term use of these drugs may lead to a number of side-effects, some of which may be particularly unfortunate for an athlete. Osteoporosis is frequently encountered during corticosteroid therapy. This serious weakening of the skeletal structure affects principally those bones with the most trabecular structure such as the ribs and vertebrae and vertebral compression fractures are a frequent complication of steroid therapy.

Long-term use of a drug which may weaken the bone structure of an individual (whose sporting activities may subject that structure to greater than normal stress) should not be contemplated lightly. Perhaps an even more significant problem, however, is the catabolic effect of glucocorticoids on skeletal muscle. Weakness of muscles in the arms and legs can occur soon after treatment is started, even with quite modest doses of these anti-inflammatory drugs. Experiments with rats have shown that very significant reductions in muscle weight can occur within 7 days of treatment. If long-term systemic steroid treatment is initiated, it must be realized that as well as the anti-inflammatory effect which will be achieved, the administered drug will largely take over the glucocorticoid role of the natural adrenal hormone.

Due to negative feedback mechanisms operating in both the hypothalamus and the anterior pituitary, the release of corticotrophin-releasing factor and adrenocorticotrophic hormone is inhibited and so the adrenal cortex is not stimulated to produce its own glucocorticoids normally. Over a period of time the adrenal cortex regresses to a state such that the adrenal gland can no longer produce sufficient quantities of glucocorticoid to support the body if the drug treatment is stopped suddenly. It is important, therefore, that following long-term treatment with a steroid, the drug must be withdrawn gradually by progressively lowering the daily dose.

Steroids are double-edged weapons in the armoury of anti-inflammatory therapy. They are powerful, anti-inflammatory drugs but they are, unfortunately, subject to a great many side-effects. The direct application of these drugs to an affected site such that a high concentration of the steroid is achieved locally but without the attainment of significant systemic levels offers the possibility of gaining the maximum usefulness of steroids with minimal toxicity. Direct application of steroids to the skin is not an entirely satisfactory method as, although they are generally well absorbed, large proportions of the active drug will be transported away by the blood and, therefore, accumulation in affected muscle or connective tissue is limited. Additionally, topical application of steroids tends to cause thinning of the skin and a slowing down of wound healing.

The local injection of a corticosteroid preparation does offer considerable advantages in the treatment of an inflammatory condition restricted to a small area of the body. Early attempts to inject steroids locally were not particularly successful as these highly soluble drugs were rapidly redistributed from the site. The development of less soluble esters of hydrocortisone and prednisolone to give fairly insoluble microcrystalline preparations which are injected as suspensions has markedly improved the successfulness of this particular technique. A single dose of an insoluble steroid preparation will provide relief for several days or even several weeks. If necessary, these local injections can be repeated to extend the period of effectiveness.

Great care must be taken when injections of steroids are given that aseptic precautions are taken to minimize the risk of the introduction of infective agents. This is especially the case where injections have to be administered intra-articularly to improve mobility and restrict damage of an affected joint. In the case of intra-articular injection, the use of a long-acting preparation such as triamcinolone hexacetonide is indicated so that repeated injections are less necessary, or at least, less frequent. Local injection of steroids is also valuable for the treatment of soft tissue injuries. They may be injected into the interior of a bursa (the fibrous sac, filled with synovial fluid which may be found between muscles or between a tendon and bone, and which facilitates frictionless movement between the surfaces that it separates), into a tendon sheath to reduce the inflammation of an affected tendon or infiltrated around the area of an inflamed ligament. Tendinitis of the elbow (tennis elbow) is a classic example of the type of injury that responds well to local corticosteroid injection.

Steroids do have the property of delaying the wound healing process. Particular care should be taken when using them in situations where extensive new tissue will have to be produced (as may be the case, for example, where a collision on the sports field has led to an open wound). In this instance the use of steroids to reduce inflammation may not be appropriate. Glucocorticoids are included in the list of prohibited classes of substances if administered orally, rectally or by intavenous or intramuscular injection. Local administration, including intra-articular injections of these antiinflammatory steroids is permissible when medically necessary but may, in some cases, require appropriate notification. The means by which these steroids exert their anti-inflammatory effects is not clear. It is probable that they have a number of activities, all of which contribute to their anti-inflammatory effects.

They have been shown to reduce the output of chemical mediators of inflammation and to inhibit the effects of mediators on the vascular endothelium, resulting in a reduction of oedema formation. They have also been shown to have a number of inhibitory actions on the responsiveness of white blood cells. They are, for example, particularly effective in reducing the activity of thymocytes, which are involved with delayed hyper sensitivity reactions. Whatever their mechanism of action, and despite the potential hazards of long-term, high-dose therapy, glucocorticoids are profoundly effective in the reduction of inflammatory reactions and their place in the treatment of sporting injuries is assured.

## Chapter 8

# Anti-anxiety Drugs and Sport

Throughout civilization and up to the present day human ingenuity has found various ways of coping with the stresses that life brings. Sometimes these entail a form of escapism into a drug-induced illusory world to eschew temporary troubles. A resort to alcohol, for example, can bring a transient euphoric uplift from pressing matters of the day. These strategies are perhaps truer today than they were in Dionysian cultures, exceptions being those countries where alcohol is taboo for religious reasons. It is generally believed that stress-induced illness is a phenomenon of contemporary urban civilization. The widespread prescription of tranquillizers and the high incidence of alcohol addiction support this view. Their impact on fitness and well-being has received scant attention.

Amongst athletes, participation in sports brings its own unique form of stress, usually before the more important contests. Though a certain amount of pre-competition anxiety is inevitable, the anxiety response varies enormously between individuals, with some people coping extremely poorly. Many find their own solutions to attenuate anxiety levels, albeit sometimes with exogenous aids. Anxiety may adversely affect performance, especially in activities highly demanding of mental concentration and steadiness of limbs. This has prompted the use of anti-anxiety drugs, although some are not permitted in many sports.

The relationship between anxiety and sport performance is first explored. The concentrates on alcohol, its metabolism in the body and its effect on the central nervous system. The interactions between alcohol and health are then considered.

Its impact on physiological responses to exercise and the uses in sport are examined next. The main 'minor' tranquillizers, the benzodiazepines and melatonin, finally, the uses and abuses of other anti-anxiety drugs are described.

## ANXIETY AND PERFORMANCE

The psychological reaction to impending sports competition is variously referred to as anxiety, arousal, stress or activation. Though these concepts are not synonymous, their relationships to performance have sufficient similarities to group them together for the present purposes. Anxiety denotes worry or emotional tension, arousal denotes a continuum from sleep to high excitement, stress implies an agent that induces strain in the organism and activation refers to the metabolic state in the 'flight or fight' reaction. Irre-spective of which concept is adopted, the effects of the biological responses on performance are generally assumed to fit an inverted-U curve. A moderate level of 'anxiety' about the forthcoming activity is deemed desirable to induce the right levels of harnessed motivation for action. The simpler the task the higher will be the level of anxiety that can be tolerated before performance efficiency begins to fall.

Although the inverted-U model is somewhat simplistic, it does illustrate that over-anxiety has a detrimental effect on the physical and psychomotor elements that comprise sports performance. In such instances anxiety-reducing strategies will have an ergogenic effect. The athlete or mentor may have to choose between mental relaxation techniques or drugs to alleviate anxiety.

There are various indices which the behavioural scientist employs in measuring anxiety in field conditions, such as sport, especially prior to competition. These include hand tremor, restlessness or other subjective estimates of 'tension', paper and pencil tests and so on. Linked to these are physiological indices which demonstrate increased sympathetic tone. These measures include muscular tension as indicated by electromyography, galvanic skin response or skin conductance and elevated concentrations of stress hormones or their metabolites in blood or in urine. These variables may be important to consider if the mechanisms by which the ergogenic or adverse effects of anxiety-reducing drugs operate are to be understood.

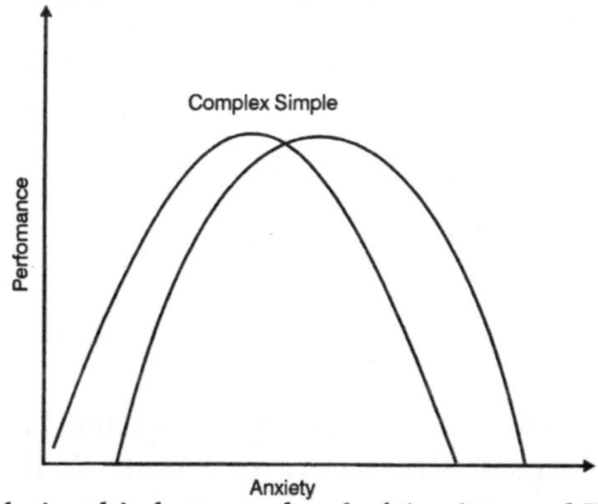


**Fig.** The Relationship between level of Anxiety and Performance Efficiency for Simple and Complex Tasks.

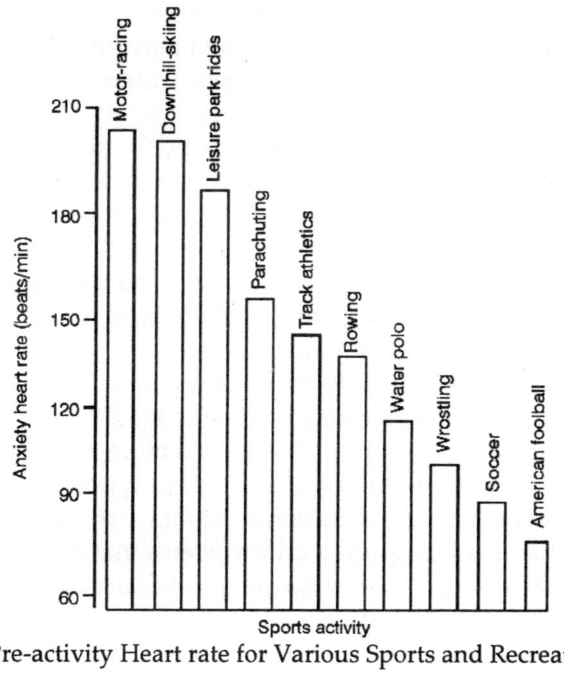


**Fig.** Pre-activity Heart rate for Various Sports and Recreations.

High levels of anxiety generally militate against

performance and so favour attempts to reduce anxiety. Anxiety level depends very much on the nature of the sport as well as on the individual concerned. Generally, high anxiety is associated with brief and high-risk activities. A league table of anxiety responses pre-start as reflected in emotional tachycardia, shows motor-racing and downhill skiing to be top of the list. Activities like para-chuting and high acceleration rides in leisure parks induce strong anxiety reactions albeit mingled with a feeling of exhilaration. In these cases heart rates have been found to correlate highly with adrenaline levels in blood and in urine. Possibly because of the practice of relaxation techniques in this group and the long duration of such games.

Professional athletes regularly subjected to situations of high psychological stress tend to adapt. At this elite level highly anxious personalities are rare. The anxiety reaction of professional soccer players, for example, is highly reproducible although there are noticeable trends. Resting heart rates in the dressing-room tend to be higher when playing at home rather than away, because players are subject to more critical scrutiny by a home audience.

Anxiety is highest in goalkeepers, for whose mistakes the team is usually punished. Players returning to the team after a spell of injury or making an initial appearance in the premier team show higher heart rates than their normal pre-match values. It is hardly surprising to find that goalkeepers are the most vulnerable members of the team to stress-related illnesses such as stomach ulcers.

Avoiding over-anxiety may be important in game players for reasons of safety. Anxiety has been found to correlate with joint and muscle injuries in soccer, the more anxious players tending to get injured most often. This supports the notion of injury proneness: the mechanism is probably lack of commitment or hesitancy in critical events that might promote injury. Traditionally, some soccer players used to take a nip of whisky immediately prior to going on to the pitch, the communal bottle being euphemistically referred to as 'team spirit'. The inhibiting effects of alcohol used to be exploited by tournament rugby players, who were not averse to drinking beer in between rounds of 'rugby sevens' competitions for example.

Obviously there is a thin line to tread between, on the one hand, reducing anxiety to enhance well-being and mental states prior to competing in sport and, on the other hand, impairing performance because of a disruption in motor co-ordination accompanying the treatment. The outcome depends on the concentrations of the drug, the timing of ingestion and the individual susceptibility to it. There are also possibilities of tolerance to the drug with chronic use or of drug dependence developing. Residual effects may carry over to the following day, affecting training or subsequent competitive performance. These aspects are now considered in the context of alcohol in sports and exercise.

## ALCOHOL

### Metabolism of Alcohol

The alcohols are a group of chemicals, most of which are toxic. The most common is ethanol or ethyl alcohol which is obtained by the fermentation of sugar. It is non-toxic, except in large and chronic doses, and has been enjoyed as a beverage for many centuries.

Ethyl alcohol is both a drug and a food, accounting for about 100 kcal (420 kJ) of energy per adult of the UK population each day. Its energy value per unit weight (kcal/g), the Atwater factor, is 7 compared with a value of 9 for fat, but this is higher than the value of 4 for both carbohydrate and protein. Wine contains about 12 per cent alcohol, and so a litre bottle will contain about 120 g with a calorific content of 840 kcal (3516 kJ). The value of alcohol as a food stuff is limited, as it is metabolized mainly in the liver and at a fixed rate of about 100 mg/kg body weight per hour. For a 70-kg individual this amounts to 7 g of alcohol hourly.

The energy is not available to active skeletal muscle and consequently it is not possible to exercise oneself to sobriety. Beer contains some electrolytes but its subsequent diuretic effect makes it less than the ideal agent of rehydration after hard physical training.

Alcohol is a polar substance which is freely miscible in water. This is due to the fact that alcohol molecules are held together by the same sort of intermolecular forces as water, namely hydrogen bonds. The alcohol molecule is also soluble in fat, it is small and has a weak charge. (As the lipophilic alkyl group becomes larger and the hydrophilic group smaller, the alcohol molecules associate preferentially with other alcohol, hydrocarbon or lipid molecules rather than water.) It easily penetrates biological membranes and can be absorbed unaltered from the stomach and more quickly from the small intestine.

The rate of absorption is influenced by the amount of food in the stomach, whether there are gas molecules in the drink and the concentration of alcohol in the drink. Absorption is quickest if alcohol is drunk on an empty stomach, if gas molecules are present in the drink and the alcohol content is high. Intense mental concentration, lowered body temperature or physical exercise tend to slow the rate of absorption.

From the gastrointestinal tract the alcohol is transported to the liver by means of the hepatic circulation. The activity of the enzyme alcohol dehydrogenase, present chiefly in the liver, governs the disappearance of alcohol from the body. In the liver, alcohol dehydrogenase converts the alcohol to acetaldehyde; it is then converted to acetic acid or acetate by aldehyde dehydrogenase. About 75 per cent of the alcohol taken up by the blood is released as acetate into the circulation. The acetate is then oxidized to carbon dioxide and water within the Krebs (or citric acid) cycle. An alternative metabolic route for acetate is its activation to acetyl co-enzyme A and further reactions to form fatty acids, ketone bodies, amino acids and steroids. Ethyl alcohol is distributed throughout the body by means of the circulatory system and enters all the body water pools and tissues, including the central nervous system. Its distribution amongst the body fluids and tissues depends on several factors, such as blood flow, mass and permeability of the tissue.

Organs such as the brain, lungs, liver and kidneys reach equilibrium quickly, whilst skeletal muscle with its relatively poorer blood supply attains its peak alcohol concentration more slowly. Initially, alcohol moves rapidly from blood into the tissues. When absorption is complete, arterial alcohol concentration falls and alcohol diffuses from the tissues into the capillary bed. This means that alcohol concentrations remain high in the peripheral venous blood due to the slower rates of metabolism and excretion.

The metabolism of alcohol in the liver is unaffected by its concentration in the blood. Some alcohol is eliminated in the breath, but this is usually less than 5 per cent of the total amount metabolized. This route is utilized in assessing safe levels for driving, forming the basis of the breathalyser tests. Small amounts of alcohol are excreted in urine and also in sweat if exercise is performed whilst drunk. Higher excretion rates through the lungs, urine and sweat are produced at high environmental temperatures and at high blood alcohol levels.

With a single drink the blood alcohol level usually peaks about 45 minutes after ingestion. This is the point where any influence on performance will be most evident. Effects on performance will generally be greater on the ascending limb than for a corresponding value on the descending limb of the blood alcohol curve; the rate of change and the direction of change of the blood alcohol concentration are more crucial factors than is the length of time alcohol is in the bloodstream. The peak is delayed about 15 minutes if strenuous exercise precedes the ingestion. This delay may be due to the reduction in blood flow to the gut that accompanies exercise, the increased blood flow to skeletal muscle and the needs of the thermoregulatory system post-exercise.

Besides the exogenous ethanol in body fluids, trace amounts of ethanol are synthesized endogenously. This endogenous ethanol is thought to arise both from bacterial fermentation in the gut and from the action of alcohol dehydrogenase on acetaldehyde derived from pyruvate. Blood levels of endogenous alcohol in the human are very low, ranging only up to about 7.5 mg in total.

Studies on alcohol and exercise are notoriously difficult to control, as most subjects will recognize the taste of the experimental treatment. Most experimenters use vodka in orange juice as the alcohol beverage: the placebo can include enough vodka to taste but not enough to produce a measurable blood alcohol concentration. Another strategy is to put a nose clip on the subject, who is then given anaesthetic throat lozenges. Subjects vary in their responses to alcohol, as does the same subject from day to day, making inferences from laboratory studies difficult.

As the effects of alcohol differ with body size, dosage is usually administered according to body weight. Effects also vary with the level of blood alcohol induced, but there is not general international agreement on acceptable maximum levels for day-to-day activities such as driving. Alcohol doses that render subjects intoxicated or drunk have little practical relevance in exercise studies and so experimental levels are usually low to moderate.

Additionally, experiments that entail alcohol ingestion should be approved by the local human ethics committee, and high alcohol dosages are unlikely to gain acceptance in experimental protocols.

## Action of Alcohol on the Nervous System

The effects of ethanol administration on central nervous tissue are due to direct action rather than to acetaldehyde, its first breakdown product. Following ethanol ingestion, very little acetaldehyde crosses the blood-brain barrier, despite elevated levels in the blood. Alcohol has a general effect on neural transmission by influencing axonal membranes and slowing nerve conductance.

The permeability of the axonal membrane to potassium and sodium is altered by the lowering of central calcium levels that results from ingesting alcohol. Alcohol has differential effects on the central neurotrans-mitters, acetylcholine, serotonin, noradrenaline and dopamine.

Alcohol blocks the release of acetylcholine and disrupts its synthesis. As a result, transmission in the central cholinergic pathways will be lowered. The ascending reticular cholinergic pathway determines the level of cortical arousal and the flow of sensory information to be evaluated by the cortex. The lowering of electro-cortical arousal reduces the awareness of stressful information and the ability of the individual to attend to specific stimuli. These de-arousing changes are reflected in alterations in the electroencephalogram with moderate to large doses of alcohol. The obvious results are impairments in concentration, attention, simple and complex reaction times, skilled performance and, eventually, short-term memory.

Alcohol decreases serotonin turnover in the central nervous system by inhibiting tryptophan hydroxylase, the enzyme essential for serotonin's biosynthesis. Activity in the neurones of serotonergic pathways is important for the experience of anxiety; output of corticosteroid hormones from the adrenal cortex increases the activity in these neurones. Alcohol has an opposing action and so may reduce the tension that is felt by the individual in a stressful situation.

An effect of alcohol is to increase activity in central noradrenergic pathways. This is transient and is followed, some hours later, by a decrease in activity. Catecholaminergic pathways are implicated in the control of mood states, activation of these pathways promoting happy and merry states. The fall in noradrenaline turnover as the blood alcohol concentration drops ties in with the reversal of mood that follows the initial drunken euphoric state. This is exacerbated by large doses of alcohol as these tend to give rise to depression.

The small alcohol molecules penetrating the blood-brain barrier stimulate the brain to release dopamine. Dopamine is regarded as a 'pleasure-related' hormone and its release is triggered in the limbic system. Stimulation of sweat glands also affects the limbic system whilst cerebral cortical activity is depressed. Pain sensors are numbed and later the cerebellum is affected, causing difficulty with balance.

Alcohol also has an effect on cerebral energy metabolism: the drug increases glucose utilization in the brain. As glucose is the main substrate furnishing energy for nerve cells, the result is that the lowered glucose level may induce mental fatigue. This will be reflected in failing cognitive functions, a decline in mental concentration and in information processing. It is unlikely that exercise, per se, will offset these effects.

The disruption of acetylcholine synthesis and release means that alcohol acts as a depressant, exerting its effect on the reticular activating system, whose activity represents the level of physiological arousal. It also has a depressant effect on the cortex: it first affects the frontal centres of the cortex before affecting the cerebellum. In large quantities it will interfere with speech and muscular co-ordination, eventually inducing sedation. In smaller doses it inhibits cerebral control mechanisms, freeing the brain from its normal inhibition. This release of inhibition has been blamed for aggressive and violent conduct of individuals behaving out of character when under the influence of alcohol.

Undoubtedly, alcohol has been a factor in crowd violence and football hooliganism on the terraces. The belief led to the banning of alcohol at football and cricket grounds in Britain in the mid-1980s. These restrictions were extended to other sporting events in the years that followed.

Clearly, alcohol will have deleterious effects on performance in sports that require fast reactions, complex decision making and highly skilled actions. It will also have an impact on hand-eye co-ordination, on tracking tasks, such as driving, and on vigilance tasks such as long-distance sailing. An effect on tracking tasks is that control movements lose their normal smoothness and precision and become more abrupt or jerky.

In vigilance tasks, some studies have shown a deterioration in performance with time on task. At high doses of alcohol, meaningful sport becomes impractical or even dangerous. Progressive effects of alcohol at different blood alcohol concentrations. An important effect of alcohol, not listed, is that it diminishes the ability to process appreciable amounts of information arriving simultaneously from two different sources.

***Table:*** Demonstrable effects of alcohol at different blood alcohol concentrations

| *Concentration level (mg/100 ml blood)* | *Effects* |
|---|---|
| 30 | Enhanced sense of well-being; retarded simple reaction time; impaired hand-eye co-ordination |
| 60 | Mild loss of social inhibition; impaired judgement |
| 90 | Marked loss of social inhibition; co-ordination reduced; noticeably 'under the influence' |
| 120 | Apparent clumsiness; loss of physical control; tendency towards extreme responses; definite drunkenness is noted |
| 150 | Erratic behaviour; slurred speech; staggering gait |
| 180 | Loss of control of voluntary activity; impaired vision |

The most frequently cited study that reported facilitatory effects of alcohol on human performance was the classic experiment of Ikai and Steinhaus. They showed that in some cases moderate alcohol doses could improve isometric muscular strength. This result was similar to that obtained by cheering and loud vocal encouragement. They explained the effect on the basis of central inhibition of the impulse traffic in the nerve fibres of the skeletal muscles during maximal effort. This depression of the inhibitory effect of certain centres in the central nervous system may allow routine practices to proceed normally without any disturbing effects. This finding has not generally been replicated when other aspects of muscular performance are considered.

## Alcohol and Health

The effects of alcohol on health are usually viewed in

terms of chronic alcoholism. Persistent drinking leads to a dependence on alcohol so that it becomes addictive. Most physicians emphasize that alcoholism is a disease rather than a vice and devise therapy accordingly. The result of excessive drinking is ultimately manifested in liver disease: cirrhosis, a serious hardening and degeneration of liver tissue, is fatal for many heavy drinkers.

Cancer is also more likely to develop in a cirrhotic liver. There is evidence of increased susceptibility to breast cancer in women who drink alcohol regularly. Cardiomyopathy or damage to the heart muscle can result from years of heavy drinking. Other pathological conditions associated with alcohol abuse include generalized skeletal myopathy, pancreatitis and cancers of the pharynx and larynx. Impairment of brain function also occurs, alco-holic psychoses being a common cause of hospitalization in psychiatric wards.

Alcohol was formerly used as an anaesthetic until it was realized that it was too dangerous to supply in large quantities for that purpose. The result of applying alcohol to living cells is that the protoplasm of the cells precipit-ates as a consequence of dehydration. Long-term damage to tissue in the central nervous system may be an unwanted outcome of habitual heavy drinking.

Heavy drinking is not compatible with serious athletics. For the athlete, drinking is usually done only in moderation, an infrequent respite from the ascetic regimens of physical training, though the odd end of season binge is customary. Nevertheless, drinking is a social convention in many sports, such as rugby, squash and water-polo, where there may be peer-group pressure to take alcohol following training or competition or at club functions. Indeed, a few high-profile footballers in the English Premier league in the late 1990s admitted to an alcohol addiction and to referral to a rehabilitation clinic for alcoholics.

The sensible athlete drinks moderately and occasionally, avoiding alcohol for at least 24 hours before competing. Hango-vers may persist for a day and disturb concentration in sports involving complex skills. The attitude of the retired athlete may be very different. If his active career is terminated abruptly and the free time that retirement releases is taken up by social drinking, the result may well be a gradual deterioration in physical condition, with body weight increasing and fitness declining. In this context, the effect of alcohol on the ex-athlete may be quite harmful.

Various institutions within sports medicine have addressed the problems of alcohol and exercise. In 1982 the American College of Sports Medicine set out a position statement on alcohol which was unequivocally against any indulgence. It underlined the adverse effects of alcohol on health and condemned the resort to alcohol by athletes. Its estimate was that there were 10 million adult problem drinkers in the United States and an additional 3.3 million in the 14-17 year age range. No evidence for any of the beneficial aspects of alcohol was mentioned.

There is a belief that moderate drinking has some positive benefits for health. Small amounts increase the flow of gastric juices and thereby stimulate digestion: in large doses, alcohol irritates the stomach lining, causing gastritis and even vomiting of blood. A national survey of lifestyles in England and Wales provided support for the view that healthy people tended to drink a little. Amongst men under 60, the likelihood of high blood pressure was found to increase with the amount of alcohol consumed. For older men and for women, light drinking was associated with lower blood pressure, even when effects due to body weight were taken into account.

It is thought also that moderate drinking provides a degree of protection against coronary heart disease. This belief may have been nurtured originally in the vineyards of France where a habitually modest consumption of wine is associated with a low incidence of heart disease. One report claimed that myocardial infarction rates were lower in moderate drinkers than in non-drinkers. A possible mechanism is the reduction in hypertension and the relaxation from business cares that drinking can bring. Moderate alcohol consumption may help haemostasis, in balancing the processes of coagulation and fibrinolysis. A link has also been shown by an increase in high-density lipoprotein cholesterol levels with moderate levels of drinking alcohol. High-density lipoprotein particles remove cholesterol from the tissues and transfer it into other particles in the blood; low-density lipoprotein, on the other hand, obtains its cholesterol from these other particles and transfers it to the tissues.

A high ratio of high-density to low-density lipoprotein fractions is generally found in well-trained endurance athletes, a low ratio being indicative of poor cardiovascular health. The effect is apparent in autopsies of alcoholics whose blood vessels are in good condition despite pathological changes in other tissues. The mechanism by which alcohol would raise the high-density lipoprotein cholesterol has not been fully explained.

It seems that for a healthy athlete in a good state of training, occasional drinking of alcohol in moderation will have little adverse effect. It is important to emphasize that any such occasional bouts of drinking should be restrained and should follow rather than precede training sessions, whose training stimulus is likely to be lowered by the soporific influence of drinking alcohol before strenuous exercise.

## ALCOHOL AND PHYSIOLOGICAL RESPONSES TO EXERCISE

Alcohol ingestion has been shown to lower muscle glycogen at rest compared with control conditions. As pre-start glycogen levels are important for sustained exercise at an intensity of about 70-80 per cent VO2max, such as marathon running, taking alcohol in the 24 hours before such endurance activities is ill-advised. Effects of alcohol on the metabolic responses to submaximal exercise seem to be small. Juhlin-Dannfelt and co-workers reported that alcohol does not impair lipolysis or free fatty acid utilization during exercise. It may decrease splanchnic glucose output, decrease the potential contribution of energy from liver gluconeogenesis, cause a more pronounced decline in blood glucose levels and decrease the leg muscle uptake of glucose towards the end of a prolonged (up to 3-hour) run.

The impairment in glucose production by the liver would

lead to an increased likelihood of hypoglycaemia developing during prolonged exercise.

Some studies have shown an increase in oxygen uptake (VO2) at a fixed submaximal exercise intensity after alcohol ingestion. This may be due to a poorer co-ordination of the active muscles as the decrease in mechanical efficiency, implied by the elevation in VO2, is not a consistent finding. Related to this is an increase in blood lactate levels with alcohol; metabolism of alcohol shunts lactate away from the gluconeogenic pathway and leads to an increase in the ratio of lactate to pyruvate. It is possible that elevated blood lactate concentrations during exercise, after taking alcohol, may reflect impairment in clearance of lactate rather than an increase in production by the exercising muscles. A failure to clear lactate would militate against performance of strenuous exercise.

Alcohol does not seem to have adverse effects on maximum oxygen consumption (VO2max) or on metabolic responses to high-intensity exercises approaching VO2max levels. At high doses (up to 200 mg per cent, i.e. 0.20 per cent blood alcohol level) it is understandable that athletes may feel disinclined towards maximal efforts that elicit VO2max values and a reduction in peak VE (minute ventilation) is usually observed. Similarly, they may be poorly motivated to sustain high-intensity exercise for as long as they would normally do. In middle-distance running events with an appreciable aerobic component, performance was found to be detrimentally affected in a dose-related manner, with increasing blood alcohol concentration (BAC) levels from 0.01 to 0.10 per cent.

Although it has not been shown conclusively that alcohol alters VE, stroke volume or muscle blood flow at submaximal exercise levels, it does decrease peripheral vascular resistance. This is because of the vasodilatory effect of alcohol on the peripheral blood vessels, which would increase heat loss from the surface of the skin and cause a drop in body temperature. This consequence would be dangerous if alcohol is taken in conjunction with exercise in cold conditions. Sampling from a hip-flask of whisky on the ski slopes may bring an immediate feeling of warmth but its disturbance of normal thermoregulation may put the recreational skier at risk of hypothermia. Frost-bitten mountaineers especially should avoid drinking alcohol as the peripheral vasodilation it induces would cause the body temperature to fall further. In hot conditions, alcohol is also inadvisable as it acts as a diuretic and would exacerbate problems of dehydration.

Studies of maximum muscular strength, in the main, show no influence of moderate to medium doses of alcohol on maximum isometric tension. Similar results apply to dynamic functions, such as peak torque measured on isokinetic dynamometers. Muscular endurance is generally assessed by requiring the subject to hold a fixed percentage of maximum for as long as possible. Here, too, the influences of moderate alcohol doses are generally found to be non-significant. This may be because the tests represent gross aspects of muscular function and, as such, are insensitive to the effects of the drug.

## ALCOHOL IN AIMING SPORTS

In aiming sports, a steady limb is needed to provide a firm platform for launching the missile at its target or to keep the weapon still. Examples of such sports are archery, billiards, darts, pistol shooting and snooker. Two pistol shooters were disqualified during the 1980 Olympics due to taking alcohol in an attempt to improve their performance. There are also aiming components in sports such as fencing and modern pentathlon, especially in the rifle-shooting discipline of the latter. In some of these sports alcohol levels are now officially monitored, whilst in others, notably darts, drinking is a conventional complement of the sport itself.

The Grand National Archery Society in the UK has not yet banned the use of alcohol in its competitions, and so alcohol is taken in small doses in the belief that it relaxes the archer, thereby steadying the hands as well as the nerves. In order to avoid fluctuating blood alcohol concentrations, the archer, like the dart thrower, tries to keep topping up the levels to prevent them reaching the descending limb of the curve.

To understand how alcohol might affect the archer, it is useful to look at the task in toto. The competitive player has to shoot three dozen arrows at each of four targets-90, 70, 60 and 50 m away-to complete a FITA (the world governing body) round. Technological improvements in bow design have helped to produce outstanding scores, leaving the gap to perfection solely due to human factors. The modern bow has two slot-in limbs which insert into a magnesium handle section and stabilizers which help to minimize vibration and turning of the bow. Muscle strength is needed to draw the bow, whilst muscle endurance is required to hold it steady, usually for about 8 seconds for each shot while the sight is aligned with the target. Deflection of the arrow tip by 0.02 mm at 90 m causes the arrow to miss the target, which gives some idea of the hand steadiness required. The archer, before release or loose, pulls the arrow towards and through the clicker (a blade on the side of the bow which aids in measuring draw length). The archer reacts to the sound of the clicker hitting the side of the bow handle by releasing the string which, in effect, shoots the arrow. Archers are coached to react to the clicker by allowing the muscles to relax; a slow reaction to the clicker is generally recognized as hesitation. This affects the smoothness of the loose and is reflected in muscle tremor causing a 'snatched loose'. For these reasons, the effects of alcohol on reaction time, arm steadiness, muscle strength and endurance, and the electromyogram of one of the arm muscles were selected as appropriate parameters to isolate and study under experimental conditions.

In the experiment, nine subjects underwent a battery of tests under four conditions: sober, placebo, 0.02 per cent blood alcohol level and 0.05 per cent blood alcohol level. The alcohol doses were administered in three equal volumes to total 500 ml over 15 minutes, 45 minutes being allowed for peak blood alcohol levels to be attained. The doses to elicit the desirable blood alcohol levels were calculated according to the formula of Hicks which was shown to be effective:

$$A = \frac{(454)(W)(R)(BAC + 0.0002)}{(0.8)(0.95)}$$

Where A=ml 95 per cent ethanol, W=body weight (lb), R=distribution coefficient of 0.765, and BAC=desired blood alcohol concentration (0.05 per cent=0.0005). A summary of the results for the performance measurement. There was no effect of alcohol on the muscular strength and muscular endurance measures; the holding time in the endurance test was about the same time as the archer normally holds the bow drawn before shooting, so that this test turned out to be reasonably realistic.

Reaction time was significantly slowed by the lower alcohol dose, a further small delay occurring at the higher blood alcohol dose. The more sensitive response of auditory reaction time to alcohol would mean, in practice, a slower reaction to the clicker and a faulty loose. Table Effects of the alcohol treatments on four experimental tests (mean ± SD).

| *Variables* | *Sober* | *Placebo* | *0.02% BAC* | *0.05% BAC* |
|---|---|---|---|---|
| Arm steadiness: Time-off-target(s) | 2.64+0.89 | 3.05±0.74 | 3.24±1.01 | 8.17+1.49 |
| Isometric strength (N) | 546±48 | 560±37 | 541±56 | 523±78 |
| Muscular endurance (s) | 11.4±2.1 | 12.0±2.5 | 12.0±2.0 | 10.8±2.0 |
| Reaction time (ms) | 211±6.5 | 209±8.5 | 223±9.6 | 226±11.2 |

Another adverse effect noted was the impairment in steadiness of the extended arm was degraded, especially at the 0.05 per cent blood alcohol level, and the variability in arm steadiness also increased with alcohol. This effect contradicts the conventional wisdom in archery and may have been due to the high load on the arm muscles when holding the bow drawn. It is possible that alcohol only operates to advantage in steadying the limb in contexts more competitive than laboratory experiments.

Some benefits were noted in the electromyographic profile. A clearer loose was observed at the low alcohol levels which would be valuable in promoting a smoother release. This was supplemented by a tendency towards a reduced tremor in the muscle with both alcohol treatments. Together, these effects would indicate a greater muscle relaxation, the tremor being normally associated with a snatched loose. These factors were partly offset by the longer holding time prior to loose induced by the alcohol treatments. The overall conclusion was that alcohol has differential effects on tasks related to archery, depending on the concentrations, the components of the performance analysed and individual reactivity to the drug.

The deleterious effects of alcohol on some aspects of archery would not apply to other aiming sports, such as darts and pistol shooting. In these the loading on the arm muscles is light, so a greater arm steadiness is likely to be induced by the drug. Another consideration is that the timing of the release is at the discretion of the subject and also is unaffected by a retarded reaction time. Reactions will have importance where the target is moving: it is noteworthy that the discipline of clay-pigeon shooting, for example, is not steeped in a history of alcohol use.

The bar-room sports, such as snooker, billiards and darts, have the alcohol industry as an adjunct to their matches. At the highest level of competition these sports are popular television spectacles. Although it is widely thought that the top performers swig large quantities of alcohol, this is not the case. Imbibition is regular but in small doses so that a moderate blood alcohol level is continually maintained (needless to say, at high blood alcohol levels, 0.15 per cent or more, whole-body stability and mental concentration would be degraded and any possible ergogenic effect would be swamped). Alcohol is not prohibited in these sports though other drugs are.

A study of the effects of elevating blood alcohol levels on tasks related to dart throwing confirmed the finding in archery. Whilst there were negative effects from the light alcohol dose (BAC 0.02 per cent) on hand-eye coordination, effects were positive for balance and dart throwing score. A higher level of 0.05 per cent led to a fall-off in performance on all tasks. Results indicated some improvement with a light dose of alcohol for dart throwers, but performance deteriorated when BAC levels reached 0.05 per cent.

In those sports that discourage alcohol for competition there is a dishar-mony in standards for what constitutes legality. (Alcohol is banned in several sports, for example modern pentathlon, fencing and shooting.) It is worthy of note that the legal limit for driving differs between countries: in Norway and Greece the limit is 50 mg/100 ml, in Ireland it is twice that level, whilst in the UK, Ireland, France and Germany the safety limit is 80 mg/100 ml.

In Sweden the legal limit is 20 mg/100 ml, whilst in Turkey any measurable alcohol level is illegal. These values refer to alcohol in blood: the corresponding (to 80 mg/100 ml) levels for breath and for urine are 35 mg/100 ml and 107 mg/100 ml, respectively. The Amateur Fencing Association in Britain has adopted the Norwegian value as its limit for competition and has incorporated dope testing at its contests since 1984. At the request of the international governing body for fencing, alcohol tests are now carried out at the Olympic Games, although it is generally accepted that alcohol abuse is not a major problem in this sport.

Testing for alcohol is also performed on competitors in the shooting event of the modern pentathlon. Here, participants are disadvantaged by any tremor in settling down to prepare for taking their shots. Although alcohol might help competitors to relax whilst taking aim, it has little ergogenic benefit in the other disciplines of the pentathlon. For various reasons, tranquillizers and beta-blocking agents have been preferred.

## ALCOHOL AND SPORTS ACCIDENTS

It has been recommended that alcohol should be outlawed prior to aquatic activities because of the potential for catastrophic accidents in the water. Alcohol is a significant factor in spinal injuries occurring in recreational water sports. In scuba diving the potential for fatal nitrogen narcosis increases at shallower depths when alcohol is consumed. Of 752 drowning victims studied in North Carolina, 53 per cent were positive for alcohol and 38 per cent had blood alcohol values of 0.10 per cent or greater.

Peak effects on motor performance following administration of alcohol are typically observed 45-60 min later, but impairment is evident for up to 3 hours after dosing.

This could render the drinker susceptible to accidents if alcohol is imbibed after sports competitions before driving the journey home. There is evidence also of impaired exercise performance the morning after a bout of nocturnal drinking, adverse effects being observed in aerobic performance. This finding has implications for the behaviour of players the night before competition or serious training.

## Benzodiazepines

Benzodiazepines, derivatives of benzodiazepine, are widely employed as tranquillizers in the population at large and have been used for calming or sedative purposes in sports. They are included in the list of drugs that may be taken by sports competitors.

There are now over two dozen benzodiazepine drugs and these form over 90 per cent of the tranquillizer market. More than 20 doses of these drugs per head of the USA population are prescribed annually, giving an idea of the vast scale of consumption.

The first benzodiazepine drug was synthesized in the mid-1950s, the best known of those that followed being Librium (chlordiazepoxide hydrochloride), introduced in the USA in 1960, and Valium (diazepam), introduced in 1963. The benzodiazepines have systematically replaced the barbiturates and the propranediol derivatives as drugs of clinical choice in treating stress and anxiety. There is little evidence that the barbiturates had a major use amongst active athletes as an ergogenic aid in the years when they were being widely prescribed, although they may have been used in more recent years.

Benzodiazepines decrease stress response indices, such as skin conductance and plasma corticosterone levels. They have been found to reduce anxiety in psychiatrie and non-psychiatric patients and have demonstrated a superiority over barbiturates in clinical conditions.

The drugs affect various neurotransmitters, the cholinergic and serotonergic effects having importance in reducing the stress response.

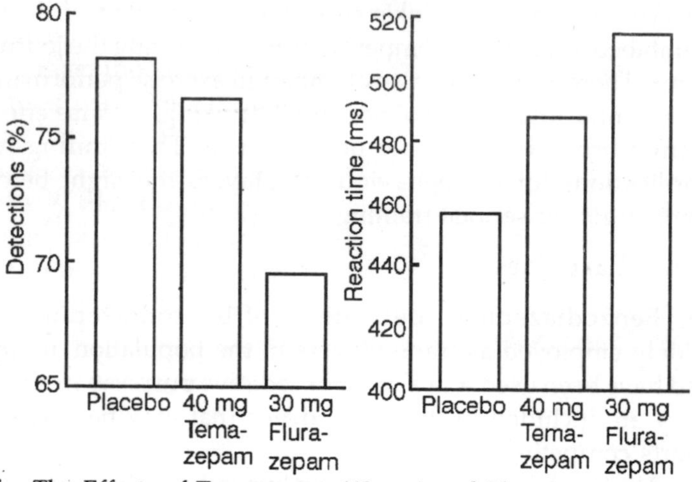


**Fig.** The Effects of Temazepam (40 mg) and Flurazepam (30 mg)

The tasks were performed the morning after nightly administration of drugs. The benzodiazepines decrease the turnover in hemispheric cholinergic neurones by blocking the release of acetylcholine. By thus lowering the activity in cholinergic pathways, the drugs should have an adverse effect on human performance. Deterioration in the detection of sensory signals and in reaction time in a rapid information-processing task with nightly doses of flurazepam and temazepam have been found the morning after taking the drugs. The carry-over effects are due to the long half-lives of these particular drugs.

Other types of performance which are affected include the rate of tapping, motor manipulation and complex co-ordination tasks, as well as real and simulated driving. The function of one particular cholinergic pathway is to trigger the release of corticotrophic-releasing factor from the hypothalamus into the pituitary blood vessels and produce a spurt of adrenocorticotrophic hormone (ACTH) from the anterior pituitary. The benzodiazepines would lower the emission of corticosteroid hormones from the adrenal cortex by affecting the ACTH release as a result of blocking cholinergic activity.

The benzodiazepines have been found to decelerate the

turnover of noradrenaline. This effect is more apparent in conditions where the noradrenaline levels have been increased by stress. This change is not the basis of the drugs' anti-anxiety action, as repeated dosing with oxazepam results in a rapid tolerance to the decrease in noradrenaline turnover, whilst the drug maintains its anti-anxiety properties. Similarly, dopamine turnover is retarded by benzodiazepines, but this effect is unrelated to the drugs' anti-anxiety properties.

The main anti-anxiety action of benzodiazepines seems to stem from the reduction in serotonergic activity which the drugs produce. Serotonergic neurones are important in the experience of anxiety, so that this feeling is attenuated by the drugs. The effects of the benzodiazepines on serotonergic neurones may be mediated by a primary action of the drugs on gamma-aminobutyric acid (GABA). (It is thought that administration of GABA has been tried by some sports competitors.) The GABA-releasing neurones are primarily inhibitory and it is possible that when these are stimulated by the benzodiazepines the release of serotonin is inhibited. The GABA system is recognized as playing a crucial role in anxiety: some anxiety-related states may be due to diminished transmission at the level of GABA receptors which are functionally linked to benzodiazepine recognition sites.

The effects of benzodiazepines on components of human performance will depend on the dosage and on the particular drug. Oxazepam, diazepam, nitrazepam, flurazepam and chlordiazepoxide are all 1,4-derivatives. Clobazam, a 1,5-benzodiazepine derivative, does not seem to impair psychomotor performance but does retain its anti-anxiety properties and so may have more applications than the others in sport and exercise contexts.

Following the bans on alcohol overuse in the modern pentathlon, athletes at the 1972 Olympic Games in Munich were found to have used benzodiazepines and other tranquillizers, such as meprobamate, as anti-anxiety agents. They were thought preferable to alcohol as they might reduce anxiety without the potential adverse effects on judgement and co-ordination associated with alcohol. Meprobamate acts as a mild tranquillizer without producing drowsiness. It is highly addictive and reduces tolerance to alcohol. The benzodiazepines are relatively safe in that they have low toxicity and few side-effects. They can induce a dependence in chronic users and severe withdrawal symptoms are experienced when patients are taken off them abruptly. They are highly dangerous when used in overdoses combined with other central nervous system depressants, such as alcohol. Benzodiazepines are banned in the sport of modern pentathlon, though not on the list banned by the International Olympic Committee (IOC).

One of the primary effects of the GABA-mediated reaction to benzodiazepines is that the drugs act as muscle relaxants. For this reason, they can be beneficial in aiding recovery from spastic-type muscle injuries. The effect is associated with a feeling of freedom from 'nerves' and tension. There are repercussions for muscle function in both submaximal and extreme efforts. Spontaneous activity of animals is reduced under the influence of these drugs. A study of alprazolam by Cabri et al. demonstrated that the effects were dependent on the dose. Maximal torque on an isokinetic dynamometer was unaffected by a low dose (0.5 mg). Moderate doses of the drug (1.5 and 3.0 mg) caused a reduction in muscle performance during brief bouts of maximal effort, both 90 and 360 minutes after ingestion.

The metabolic effects were reflected in a decrease in amplitude and integrated electromyogram, but these effects were reduced after 360 minutes. It was thought that GABA-ergic activity induced alterations both in central nervous system and in peripheral (neuromuscular) receptor sites for benzodiazepines. Different benzodiazepine drugs vary in their pharmacokinetic profiles and so their influence on muscle performance may also be variable. For this reason, Zinzen et al. compared the effects of therapeutic doses of flunitrazepam (plasma half-life of 31 hours) and triazolam (half-life of 8 hours) on performance, utilizing an isokinetic dynamometer. No hangover effects were noted after an 8-hour sleep with triazolam; in contrast, flunitrazepam was shown to impair muscle force production after the night's sleep and subjects were reported as having a 'sleepy impression' throughout the following day. Various stimulants, including caffeine, have been used to offset the depressant effects of benzodiazepines on psychomotor skills. Caffeine interacts with the GABA-benzodiazepine system and so may reverse some adverse effects of these tranquillizers. Collomp et al. showed that moderate benzodiazepine intake (1 mg of lorazepam) significantly impaired performance on an all-out exercise test over 30 seconds. Moderate caffeine intake (250 mg of caffeine in combination with 1 mg of lorazepam) antagonized the metabolic but not the performance effects of the tranquillizer.

Diazepam is frequently prescribed in the treatment of muscle spasm. As doses used for relaxation of skeletal muscle, the drug could cause drowsiness and impair intellectual as well as motor function. Diazepam would generally be used on a short-term basis for treating muscle spasm due to injury. Consequently it does not entail withdrawal symptoms when treatment is complete.

The effects of benzodiazepines on sustained exercise performance are poorly documented. In the resting normal human, coronary blood flow is increased by 22.5 per cent by diazepam but more so (73 per cent) in persons with coronary artery disease. Whether the drugs are of benefit in the treatment of angina associated with effort is unknown.

Barbiturates and sedatives have long been used in sleeping pills. Such a use, to facilitate the sleep of athletes the night before competition, is likely to be counterproductive because of a residual de-arousing effect the following day. The 'hangover' effect of benzodiazepines was found to be greater for flurazepam (30 mg) than for temazepam (40 mg). Although the former produced better sleep, it resulted in lowered clear-headedness on waking and impaired performance on a rapid visual information-processing task.

The 'hangover' effect of sleeping tablets, including benzodiazepines, is likely to disturb complex skills more than simple motor tasks performed early the following day, and, depending on the sport, an increase in errors may promote a higher risk of injury. Alcohol can compound the adverse effects of other drugs on motor performance tasks. Attention and reaction time tasks are impaired by a combination of temazepam and ethanol in doses which may not cause impairment when each is given alone. Subjects tend to be unaware of their reduced performance capabilities when taking these drugs in combination. There are likely to be increases also in injury risk. Of 402 victims of ski accidents, 20 per cent were positive for alcohol, 8.5 per cent had taken benzodiazepines and 2.5 per cent were positive for both drugs. Subjects positive for both tended to be older than the other persons examined.

Benzodiazepines have been thought to help in adjusting circadian rhythms following time-zone transitions because of their promotion of sleep. Reilly et al. found temazepam had no effect in combating jet-lag in British athletes travelling over five time-zones to the USA. There was no effect on the rate of adjustment to the new time-zone, either in core temperature, performance measures or subjective symptoms. The ease of sleeping following travelling westwards and arriving in the evening local time probably rendered any sleep elixir superfluous in these circumstances. Low doses of benzodiazepines may benefit shift workers who have difficulty in sleeping during the day after a nocturnal shift. In a study of simulated shift work, Wesnes and Warburton found that 10-20 mg doses of temazepam helped daytime sleep without detrimental residual effects on subsequent information processing.

The circadian or 24-hour rhythm in arousal may have implications for the pharmacological effects of anti-anxiety drugs. The optimum dosage of drugs affecting the nervous system differs with the time of day at which they are administered. The barbiturate dose that is safe in the evening may have exaggerated effects in early morning. The same is true for alcohol and this is reflected in social drinking habits: usually only alcoholics drink before breakfast and in the late morning. Alcohol taken at lunch time has a much more detrimental effect on psychomotor performance than if taken in the evening. The diurnal variation in responses to benzodiazepines and the implications this has for the dosage at different times of day for effective pre-contest tranquillization does not seem to have been the subject of any serious research attention.

## Melatonin

Melatonin is a hormone produced by the pineal gland. The main claims for its use have been as a hypnotic to aid sleep and as a chronobiotic to counteract jet-lag. It has antioxidant properties and so has been promoted to combat free radicals which are produced during exercise. It is widely available in the USA but is not licensed for use in the UK and some other European countries. In countries where it is openly available, it has been used with the aim of reducing stress.

Melatonin has a lowering effect on body temperature, probably due to its vasodilatory effects on peripheral blood vessels. Its chronobiotic effect depends on the timing of the dose and whether the intention is to shift the timing of the body clock forwards or backwards, its so-called phase-response curve. Bright light opposes the action of melatonin, inhibiting its production. Secretion would normally start at about 21:00 hours or after onset of darkness and ends at around 08:00 hours. The normal circadian rhythm is disrupted on rapid time-zone transitions and has led to the use of melatonin to hasten the adjustment of the body clock to the new time-zone.

Like benzodiazepines, melatonin can have unpredictable side-effects. These include fuzzy head, sleepiness, disrupted concentration and increased feelings of fatigue. There are possible allergic reactions in some individuals. For these reasons the British Olympic Association has advised caution among its athletes and officials considering using melatonin. In promoting adjustment of the body clock following long-haul flights, behavioural and natural means-such as light, exercise, social activity, sleeping/waking-were preferred. In the typical circumstances which travellers experience, melatonin appears to be ineffective.

The hypnotic effects of melatonin are reflected in the advice not to drive after ingesting this substance. Auditory vigilance, reaction time and feelings of vigour have all been adversely affected after ingesting melatonin during the day. Deterioration in muscle strength or performance in a 4-km cycle time-trial the morning after taking melatonin prior to going to bed. There was little evidence of an improvement in sleep quality among the athletes.

## Marijuana

Marijuana is obtained from the hemp plant Cannabis saliva. It contains the compound tetrahydrocannabinol which accounts for its psychological effects. These include a sedating and euphoric feeling of well-being and relaxation, with a sensation of sleepiness. Balance may be disturbed; aggression and motivation to perform may be blunted. Maximum muscular strength is reduced, probably because of the reduced drive towards all-out effort.

Largely because of its promotion of happy and euphoric mood states, marijuana has been prominent amongst the drugs of abuse, notably by youngsters and college students in the USA and Europe. It was the main recreational drug used by late adolescents and young adults in the 1970s. A report of the US Department of Health and Human Services, Student Drug Use in America 1975 to 1980, claimed that nearly one-third of students had tried marijuana before entering high school. This background of experience with the drug might explain its popularity amongst young athletes as a mode of release from tension during the competitive season. Like alcohol it is included in the IOC's list of prohibited substances as subject to certain restrictions.

In recent years the IOC has introduced a cut-off level for carboxy-THC of 15 ng/ml. Statistics from IOC-accredited laboratories indicate an increasing number of positive tests for marijuana since 1994 when 75 positive results were reported. It is likely that this trend reflects an increased use of the drug in society as a whole. The positive result from Ross Rebagliati at the 1998 Winter Olympic Games in Nagano was attributed by the athlete to passive smoking. Clearly elite athletes are equally exposed to the leisure-drug culture as are non-athletic young members of society. Persistent marijuana smoking is incompatible with serious athletic training. The single-mindedness of the athlete will be disturbed by the demotivating influence of the drug. A few cigarettes of marijuana may cause minor changes in personality, while high doses can induce hallucinations, delusions and psychotic-like symptoms. The major abuse of marijuana has been by collegiate games teams, playing basketball and football, in the USA. The practice of smoking marijuana is generally condemned by athletic trainers and coaches in that country.

The active ingredient in marijuana is 1-5-9-tetrahydrocannabinol (THC). About 60 to 65 per cent of the THC in a marijuana cigarette is absorbed through the lungs when it is smoked. Effects of drug action are noted within 15 minutes of smoking and last for 3 hours or so. The primary effects are produced by changes in central nervous system function. Motivation for physical effort is decreased and motor co-ordination, short-term memory and perception are impaired. Chronic marijuana abuse has been found to include decreased circulating testosterone levels amongst its toxic effects. In addition to the psychological effects, marijuana induces tachycardia, bronchodilation and an increase in blood flow to the limbs. The bronchodilation effect does not lead to substantial alteration of the respiratory pattern during exercise.

A pre-exercise increase of heart rate by 25 beats/minute is sustained during exercise up to about 80 per cent of maximal effort. This means that maximal heart rate is attained at a lower intensity during a graded exercise test and the maximal work capacity is decreased after marijuana smoking. In another study, a general decrement in standing steadiness, simple and complex reaction times, and psychomotor skills was observed following administration of 215 mg/kg of the active ingredient of marijuana.

## Nicotine

The tobacco leaf, Nicotiana tabacum, is the source of the cigarettes on which the massive tobacco industry is based. As the tobacco burns it generates about 4000 different compounds, including carbon monoxide (CO), ammonia, hydrogen cyanide, many carcinogens, DDT and tar.

Carbon monoxide reduces the oxygen transport capacity of the blood by combining with haemoglobin (Hb) and so takes the place of oxygen in the bloodstream, adversely affecting aerobic exercise performance. The affinity of CO for Hb is 230 times that of oxygen. Tobacco smoke contains about 4 per cent CO; smoking 10-12 cigarettes a day results in a blood COHb level of 4.9 per cent, 15-25 a day raises the value to 6.3 per cent, whilst 30-40 each day takes the level to 9.3 per cent. Adverse effects are noticeable only during physical exertion, and after smoking it may take 24 hours or more for blood CO levels to return to normal. The smoke also paralyses the cilia in the respiratory passages so that their filtering becomes ineffective and the individual is more susceptible to respiratory tract infections.

The anti-smoking argument is centred around the links between smoking and cancer. Another strong link has been shown between smoking and hardening of the peripheral arteries and deterioration of the circulation to the limbs. The result can be a need for amputation of the affected limb. Other long-term health hazards associated with heavy smoking are acceleration of coronary atherosclerosis, pulmonary emphysema and cerebral vascular disease.

About 30 per cent of the adult population throughout the world smoke cigarettes and it is likely that double this number have sampled cigarettes at some time or another. As passive inhalation of smoke by non-users of tobacco-especially in crowded public places-has similar effects to those in smokers, smoking in public facilities is now restricted in many countries. About 20 per cent of the smoke exhaled can be recirculated in passive inhalation. The psychological and addictive effects of smoking are attributable to nicotine. Smokers report that cigarettes help them to relax, and the intensity of smoking increases at times of stress. They also report that smoking has a tranquillizing effect when they are angry. These influences on subjective states do not tally with the neurochemical and physiological responses to nicotine.

Nicotine is a cholinergic agonist and so by acting as a brain stimulant is likely to enhance arousal. In this respect it differs from alcohol and the benzodiazepines. There is a secondary rise in plasma corticosteroids, and an increase in central release of noradrenaline and in urinary catecholamine output. These changes are normally associated with the stress response, so that the relaxing characteristics of nicotine present a paradox.

A few theories attempting to resolve this conflict were reviewed by Wesnes and Warburton, though none fitted all the experimental evidence satisfactorily. They argued that it is the action of nicotine on cholinergic pathways controlling attention that reduces stress by enabling individuals to concentrate more efficiently.

Neurotic individuals, who comprise the majority of smokers, are helped by the drug to filter out distracting thoughts; this enables them to perform more effectively, increasing their self-confidence in the process.

Smokers tend to experience stress when trying to give up cigarettes. For this reason, games players and other athletes who smoke pre-competition need astute counselling in attempting to overcome the habit. This would be best done during non-critical periods of the week and the pre-match smoking could be replaced unobtrusively by behavioural techniques of relaxation.

However, resort to smoking may be easily replaced by an increase in snacks between meals, leading to unwanted weight gain. This occurs because the appetite centre in the brain is released from the depressant effect that smoking has on it. This problem will be greatest in the casual recreationist whose energy expenditure during physical activity will generally be low.

Quite apart from the effects on health and on human performance, smoking may also have repercussions for sports injury, particularly under conditions of cold. An acute effect of smoking is peripheral vasoconstriction which decreases blood flow to the limbs. For this reason, the frost-bitten climber should avoid any temptation to smoke until after recovery through hospitalization where alternative therapies are ensured.

Clearly cigarette smoking has few advocates in sport and the sports sciences. Advertising of cigarettes is prohibited in some Scandinavian countries and top athletes are frequently prominent in anti-smoking campaigns. Sports associations that enjoy sponsorship from tobacco companies have come under pressure to find alternative benefactors. Smoking is rare amongst elite athletes, so that there are few models for youngsters taking up smoking to cite as examples. Those sports stars that do smoke might ultimately benefit from adopting alternative strategies to ease their troubled minds at times of emotional stress.

## Beta Blockers

Sympathetic adrenergic nerve fibres are classified according to their alpha and beta receptors. Effects of these receptors are sometimes contradictory. In the blood vessels of muscle and skin, α-adrenergic receptors cause vasoconstriction, whereas β-receptors induce vasodilation. The beta β-receptors are further divided into β1 - and β2 -categories according to the responses to sympathomimetic drugs. Functions of β1 -receptors include cardiac acceleration and increased myocardial contractility; β2 -receptors cause bronchodilation and glycogenesis. The action of these receptors is blocked by the activities of inhibitory drugs, the so-called beta blockers. These include, for example, atenolol, a cardioselective beta blocker with selectivity for β1 - adrenoceptors; propranolol, which blocks both types of β-receptors, and labetalol which is a combined alpha and beta blocker.

Besides decreasing heart rate and myocardial contractility, the beta-blocking agents also reduce cardiac output, stroke volume and mean systemic arterial blood pressure. These effects explain the use of beta blockade in hypertension and in individuals with poor coronary health. Because of the effects on the circulation, beta blockade in clinical doses reduces maximal oxygen uptake and endurance time in normal individuals, but increases maximal work capacity in patients with angina pectoris. At submaximal exercise levels a decrease in heart rate and contractility is balanced by a decrease in coronary blood flow and an increased duration of myocardial contraction. The fall in exercise heart rate is not matched by a corresponding drop in perceived exertion rating, so that the usual close correlation between these variables is dissociated by beta blockade.

The effects of beta blockers on metabolism have implications for the performance of submaximal exercise. By inhibiting the enzyme phosphorylase, beta blockade may decrease the rate of glycogenolysis in skeletal muscle. Breakdown of liver glycogen is also likely to be inhibited, so that in sustained exercise blood glucose levels may decline. This fall is noted with propranolol but is not so evident with atenolol or metoprolol, two cardioselective beta blockers. Kaiser showed that jogging was markedly influenced only by propranolol at the low dose of 40 mg: at doses of 80 mg and above, atenolol had a similar adverse effect. Selective beta blockade inhibits lipolysis, which may reduce the availability of free fatty acids as a substrate for prolonged exercise and cause an earlier onset of fatigue.

The effect of beta blockade on short-term high-intensity performance was examined by Rusko et al.. The subjects performed a range of anaerobic tasks after taking the beta blocker oxprenolol, and results were compared with performances after being given an inert placebo. The drug had no effect on isometric strength of leg extension, vertical jumping and stair running. Power output over 60 seconds on a cycle ergometer was reduced under the influence of the drug, whilst peak blood lactate and heart rates were also decreased. It seems that the beta blocker caused a reduction in anaerobic capacity as well as in heart rate.

Use of beta blockers has implications for thermoregulation if exercise is conducted in the heat. Gordon et al. showed that a non-selective beta blocker (propranolol) produced greater sweating than did a β1 -selective blocker (atenolol). In this study, both drugs produced equivalent reductions in exercise tachycardia, a similar decrease in skin blood flow and a similar rise in rectal temperature. The authors suggested that β1 - selective adrenoceptor blockers should be the preferred therapy during prolonged physical activity when adequate fluid replacement cannot be guaranteed.

The findings indicated an increased need for persons treated with propranolol to stick to a strict fluid replacement regimen during sustained exercise.

Another consideration is whether the physiological adaptations to a fitness training programme are altered by the use of beta blockers. Propranolol, even in low doses of 80 mg daily, does blunt the effects of exercise training in normal individuals. At higher doses of 160-320 mg/day, this impairment is more pronounced. The apparent mechanism is a prevention of the normal peripheral circulatory and metabolic responses to exercise. Although beta blockade permits patients with angina to exercise more easily, the chronic effects of physical training in patients with ischaemic heart disease may still be attenuated. Indeed, Powles considered that the many physiological effects of beta blockade meant that for each patient there may be an optimal dosage. This optimal point is that at which adverse effects on the functioning of the left ventricle, the myocardial perfusion and metabolism did not outweigh the benefits associated with decreased heart rate.

Beta blockers cross the blood-brain barrier to varying extents, depending on their lipid solubility; for example, propranolol does so to a greater degree than atenolol. Their anti-anxiety effect may not necessarily be centrally mediated. The suppression of cardiac activity which would result in a reduction in the afferent information from the heart may be the cause. Inhibition of the β-receptors, through which glycogenolysis is stimulated by adrenaline and lactic acid production is increased, is an alternative mechanism. Low levels of lactic acid tend to be associated with a state of relaxation, free from anxiety.

On balance, however, the evidence favours the interpretation that the anti-anxiety effects of these drugs are due to direct action within the central nervous system. As beta-blocking agents are not addictive they tend to be preferred over the benzodiazepines and alcohol in combating anxiety. They attenuate emotional tachycardia, limb tremor and unpleasant manifestations of anxiety, such as palmar sweating, pre-competition. These drugs have proved effective in reducing anxiety in students undergoing oral examinations, in public speakers and in musicians liable to 'stage-fright'. High-risk sports, such as ski-jumping, motor-racing and bobsleighing, provide especially suitable contexts for their use. Undesirable effects might be produced by beta blockers in athletes suffering from asthma and in individuals with reduced cardiac function.

The beta blockers have been banned by the International Shooting Union as they are believed to be of potential use to marksmen in reducing anxiety before competitions and enhancing performance. Nevertheless, they were repeatedly used by many competitors in shooting events at the 1984 Olympic Games (and to a lesser extent at the subsequent Games), being prescribed by team physicians for health reasons. Similar practices by top professional snooker players were disclosed at the 1987 World Championship. They are unlikely to be used in endurance events where the aerobic system is maximally or near-maximally taxed. They would have an ergogenic effect in the shooting discipline of the modern pentathlon, an event in which they have allegedly been used for a steadying influence before shooting.

The use of beta blockers in selected sports was reflected in the IOC Medical Commission's decision to test for beta blockers only in the biathlon, bob sled, figure-skating, luge and ski-jump competitions at the 1988 Winter Olympic Games in Calgary. In the 1988 Summer Olympic Games in Seoul, and the 1992 Summer Games in Barcelona, the IOC Medical Commission tested for beta blockers in the archery, diving, equestrian, fencing, gymnastics, modern pentathlon, sailing, shooting and synchronized swimming events only.

Studies of the effects of beta blockers on pistol shooters suggest that they are mainly of benefit to the less competent and less experienced shooters, as well as those most anxious prior to competition.

A study of the British national pistol squad found that significant improvement in shooting scores was restricted to slow-fire events, the ergogenic effect being slightly greater for an 80 mg dose than for 40 mg of oxprenolol.

The effect of a 40 mg dose of oxprenolol was matched by an effect of alcohol equivalent to a half pint (284 ml) of beer. There appeared to be a substantial placebo effect which applied equally to alcohol and beta blockers.

# Index


## A

Absorption 4, 5, 16, 17, 27, 82, 104, 263, 264, 281, 295, 296
Abuse in Sport 61, 63, 67, 89, 102, 120, 155, 158, 199, 218, 243, 252
Abuse of Acth 231
Action of Alcohol 281, 282
Acute and Chronic 248
Administration and Supply 222
Alcohol and Sports 294
Anaemia 172, 266
Androgenic Anabolic 50, 51, 52, 53, 54, 55, 163
Androgenic Effects 169
Anti-Anxiety Drugs 275, 276, 300
Anticholinergic Drugs 135
Anticholinergics 142
Attitudes Towards 61, 62

## B

Behavioural Effects 82, 220
Benzodiazepines 58, 276, 295, 296, 297, 298, 299, 300, 301, 305, 309
Beta Blockers 11, 30, 41, 57, 58, 125, 306, 307, 308, 309, 310
Biochemistry 16, 165, 167, 198, 203, 232
Biosynthesis 164, 174, 194
Blood Doping 30, 37, 42, 44, 56, 74
Blood Volume 173, 199, 200, 241
Bronchodilator Drugs 130

## C

Caffeine 191, 102, 103, 104, 105, 106, 107, 108, 109, 110, 111, 112, 113, 114, 115, 116, 117, 118, 119, 134, 135, 157, 158, 160, 299
Caffeine Combinations 119
Carbohydrate 19, 20, 21, 22, 98, 99, 105, 106, 110, 111, 117, 232, 279
Carcinomas 203
Cardiovascular 131, 135, 141, 149, 150, 151, 156, 163, 198, 199, 202, 288
Central Nervous 1, 16, 27, 47, 76, 88, 131, 135, 153, 155, 158, 160, 264, 275, 280, 282, 283, 285, 286, 298, 303, 309
Changes in the Microcirculation 239, 245, 247
Classes of Drugs Subject 41, 43, 58, 60

Classes of Medicinal Products 17
Complex Drug Reactions 15
Corticosteroids 25, 43, 55, 59, 126, 127, 128, 129, 131, 141, 143, 158, 206, 231, 270, 305
Creatine 21, 22, 30, 117
Cycling 33, 34, 38, 42, 56, 74, 84, 138, 156, 157, 158, 176, 177, 230

## D

Definition 1, 17, 19, 30, 31, 36, 37, 38, 39, 44, 45, 66, 68, 71, 134, 237
Demulcents 144, 159, 160, 161
Detection of Acth 231
Detection of Hgh Abuse 229
Diclofenac 256, 263, 265, 268, 269
Doping Classes and Methods 39, 43
Doping Methods 42, 43, 68
Dosage Forms For Drug 3
Drugs and the Law 17
Drugs with Sedative Action 57
Duration of Nsaid Treatment 267

## E

Educational and Social 214
Effect of Amphetamines 77
Effect of Exercise 9, 143
Effects of Caffeine 106, 107, 108, 109, 110, 112, 115, 116, 118, 119
Effects on Adipose Tissue 222
Epidemiology 123, 180
Exercise and Asthma 136
Expectorants 144, 159, 161
Extent of Usage 178

## F

Fertility 203, 204

## G

General Side-Effects 173, 198
Ginseng 21, 153
Glucose Regulation 228
Glycoprotein Hormones 219
Growth Hormone 9, 21, 41, 53, 55, 56, 191, 193, 219, 220, 225
Gynaecological 171
Gynaecomastia 53, 204, 205, 234

## H

Human Growth 9, 219, 220, 225
Hypertension 27, 53, 80, 89, 105, 148, 199, 287, 306

## I

Ibuprofen 253, 256, 263, 264, 268
Indirect Consequences 213
Indomethocin 264
Insulin 1, 53, 110, 146, 185, 191, 193, 206, 219, 220, 221, 223, 224, 228, 232
Ioc Regulations 5, 18, 25, 26, 50, 152, 198, 234

## J

Jaundice 173

## L

L-Carnitine 22, 23, 30
Legitimate the rapeutic 23, 31, 61

Leucocytes in Inflammation 245
Leukotriene Antagonists 129, 140, 142
Local Anaesthetics 43, 58, 59, 160
Long-Term Risks of Anabolic 213
Luteinizing Hormone 40, 233, 235

## M

Management of Asthma 124, 125, 131
Marijuana 18, 25, 26, 29, 38, 43, 302, 303
Mast Cell Stobilizers 140
Mechanism of Action 1, 2, 106, 111, 255, 256, 257, 259, 274
Melatonin 276, 301, 302
Methyl Xanthines 102, 107, 134, 135, 141
Minimize Cooling 139
Mode of Action 27, 29, 81, 128, 135, 162, 167

## N

Nandrolone 19, 41, 42, 164, 170, 172, 175, 178, 179, 194, 195, 196, 197, 198, 200, 207, 233, 234
Naproxen 256, 261, 262, 263, 264, 265
Narcotic Analgesics 16, 18, 25, 26, 27, 28, 40, 49, 50, 144
Non-Drug Treatment 125, 138
Nsaids in Sports Injury 260, 268

## O

Oedema 124, 128, 129, 173, 241, 251, 257, 262, 270, 274
Oedema 173
Other Sympathomimetics 88

## P

Pathophysiology 122, 123, 137
Performance Continuation 23, 24
Precursors, Nandrolone 194
Prevalence of Hcg Abuse 234
Protein Anabolism 171, 192
Proteins and Amino Acids 20
Proteolytic Enzymes 248, 256, 269

## R

Rationale 36, 46, 177, 232
Recommendations 160, 161, 177
Recreation/Social 26
Release of Human 219
Replacement the Rapy 171
Respiratory Tract 59, 124, 138, 143, 159, 160, 161, 304
Rofecoxib and Celecoxib 267

## S

Salt and Water Retention 199
Sex-Related Side-Effects 203
Short-Term Endurance 116
Side-Effects Associated 13, 14, 36, 52, 83, 227
Side-Effects in Athletes 101
Side-Effects of Drugs 13, 14
Sodium Cromoglycate 127, 140, 141
Sources, Supply and Control 174
Specific Actions 205
Sports Medicine 1, 287

Stacking 177, 178
Stepping Down 127
Stimulants 25, 26, 32, 34, 40, 47, 49, 51, 76, 77, 78, 88, 115, 119, 120, 132, 133, 148, 154, 155, 156, 158, 179, 299
Strange Case of Clenbuterol 192

## T

Testosterone Family 164
Tolerance and Dependence 28, 79
Toxicity 14, 15, 16, 23, 27, 53, 80, 101, 102, 141, 214, 264, 270, 273, 298
Treatment of Coughs 143, 144, 147, 160
Treatment of Sporting 251, 262, 274
Trigger Factors 124, 125, 136

## U

Use and Abuse 32, 67

## V

Ventricular Function 200
Vitamins 19, 20

## W

Warm-Up 139

## X

Xanthines 102, 104, 107, 134, 135, 141, 144, 160